BEYOND BURNOUT

BEYOND BURNOUT

Stress, Resilience, and Organisational Support in Healthcare

BY

FILOMENA RIEMMA
University of Naples Parthenope, Italy

emerald PUBLISHING

United Kingdom – North America – Japan – India
Malaysia – China

Emerald Publishing Limited
Emerald Publishing, Floor 5, Northspring, 21-23 Wellington Street, Leeds LS1 4DL

First edition 2026

British Library Cataloguing in Publication Data
A catalogue record for this book is available from the British Library

ISBN: 978-1-80686-898-8 (Print)
ISBN: 978-1-80686-897-1 (Online)
ISBN: 978-1-80686-899-5 (Epub)

Printed and bound by CPI Group (UK) Ltd, Croydon, CR0 4YY

CONTENTS

INTRODUCTION

Healthcare is often described as a vocation of service, compassion and technical excellence. Yet behind the inspiring stories of healing and innovation lies a stark and enduring reality: healthcare work is profoundly stressful. From emergency departments to community clinics, from surgeons to home-care nurses, professionals confront relentless demands, complex ethical decisions and an unceasing pressure to balance efficiency with humanity. Stress in healthcare is not an occasional disruption; it is a defining characteristic of the sector, one that shapes not only the lives of those who provide care but also the outcomes of those who receive it.

The COVID-19 pandemic crystallised this reality for the world. Images of exhausted clinicians, overwhelmed hospitals and frontline staff pushed beyond endurance revealed the fragility of healthcare systems and the human cost of chronic stress. Yet as striking as those images were, they did not reveal a new phenomenon. They magnified trends that had been present for decades: workforce shortages, rising demand from ageing populations, bureaucratic inefficiencies and a culture that too often normalises burnout as a badge of honour. The pandemic was not a rupture but an accelerant, forcing healthcare systems to confront questions that had long been postponed: How can professionals be expected to deliver safe and compassionate care when their own well-being is systematically undermined? How can healthcare organisations sustain resilience when the very people who constitute their core are stretched to breaking point?

This book is an attempt to address those questions by bringing together theory, evidence and practice. It argues that stress in healthcare must be understood not merely as an individual problem to be solved through better coping strategies but as a *systemic condition* shaped by organisational culture, leadership practices, workforce planning and policy environments. While individuals can and do develop resilience, the burden of stress cannot be left on their shoulders alone. Healthcare organisations and systems bear a responsibility to create environments that protect and sustain well-being. Indeed, as the evidence consistently demonstrates, staff well-being and patient care are not separate priorities but *two sides of the same coin*: when professionals thrive, patients are safer, outcomes improve and organisations are more sustainable.

The book is structured in four parts. *Part I* sets the stage by examining healthcare as a uniquely high-pressure environment, tracing the consequences of stress for professionals, patients and organisations. *Part II* reviews classic and contemporary theories of stress, showing how models such as the Transactional Model of Stress and Coping, the Demand–Control framework and the Job Demands–Resources model provide essential insights but also require adaptation to capture the unique realities of healthcare. *Part III* builds on these insights, rethinking stress theories through the lens of healthcare evidence, highlighting phenomena such as moral distress, emotional labour and collective resilience. *Part IV* looks forward, asking what it will take to move from crisis-driven responses to long-term sustainability. It explores the alignment of leadership, policy and workforce strategies and reflects on the future of work and care in a world shaped by demographic shifts, digitalisation and global health crises.

The central argument running through the book is that stress in healthcare is *both a threat and an opportunity*. Left unaddressed, it erodes well-being, undermines patient safety and destabilises healthcare systems. Confronted honestly and strategically, it can become a catalyst for innovation, solidarity and systemic reform. Healthcare systems that take stress seriously – measuring it, addressing its causes and embedding support into their structures – are not only more humane but also more effective and resilient.

This book is written for multiple audiences. For *academics*, it offers theoretical contributions by integrating sector-specific insights from healthcare into broader models of stress and resilience. For *managers and leaders*, it provides evidence-based practices and interventions that can be implemented to reduce stress and enhance well-being. For *policymakers*, it underscores the urgency of embedding workforce sustainability into health policy and governance. For *healthcare professionals themselves*, it aims to validate lived experiences and highlight pathways towards more supportive and sustainable systems of care.

In bringing these perspectives together, the book aspires to bridge the gap between theory and practice, research and policy, and individual coping and systemic reform. Stress in healthcare cannot be solved by any one actor alone; it requires *collective responsibility* and *integrated action*. The insights presented here are therefore not a final word but an invitation: to rethink assumptions, to challenge cultures of overwork and silence and to imagine healthcare systems that protect those who care as much as those who are cared for.

The chapters that follow build a case for this transformation, combining empirical evidence, theoretical innovation and practical recommendations. They show that while the pressures of healthcare are unlikely to diminish, the way we respond to them can and must change. The future of healthcare depends not on the absence of stress but on our ability to *transform stress into resilience*, creating systems that are sustainable, compassionate and just.

Part I

UNDERSTANDING PRESSURE IN HEALTHCARE

Healthcare is often described as one of the most demanding professions in the world. The stakes are uniquely high: decisions must be taken quickly, resources are often scarce and the margin for error is minimal because lives are directly at risk. Over the past decades, the pressures on healthcare professionals have intensified rather than diminished. Global health crises such as the COVID-19 pandemic revealed vulnerabilities that were long present in hospitals, clinics and community care settings. At the same time, structural issues – staff shortages, ageing populations, increasing patient expectations and the rapid introduction of new technologies – have created a climate where pressure has become a permanent condition rather than an occasional challenge.

This part of the book sets the stage for understanding why healthcare is such a distinctive environment for studying stress and coping. While stress is a universal human experience, its contours in healthcare are sharper, more complex and often less forgiving. The combination of emotional labour, ethical dilemmas and constant exposure to suffering generates forms of strain that go beyond traditional workplace stressors. Understanding these pressures requires us to look not only at the individual professional but also at the organisational and systemic contexts in which care is delivered.

The chapters that follow pursue two complementary goals. Chapter 1 provides a panoramic view of the 'perfect storm' that characterises stress in healthcare, weaving together structural challenges and the lived experiences of professionals. Chapter 2 then maps the theoretical frameworks that scholars and practitioners have developed to make sense of stress and coping. Taken together, these chapters provide the conceptual foundation for the rest of the book: they explain not only *what* pressures healthcare workers face but also *how* we can interpret and address them through theory, research and practice.

1

THE PERFECT STORM: STRESS AND COMPLEXITY IN HEALTHCARE

ABSTRACT

This chapter conceptualises healthcare as a paradigmatic high-pressure work environment, characterised by structural, emotional and organisational complexity. Drawing on interdisciplinary literature from organisational psychology, health management and occupational health, it argues that stress in healthcare is not an episodic phenomenon but a defining and persistent feature of contemporary healthcare systems. This chapter first examines the intrinsic sources of pressure in healthcare work, including life-and-death decision-making, chronic understaffing, long working hours, emotional labour and role conflict within increasingly complex organisational settings. Particular attention is given to the COVID-19 pandemic as a critical stress test that amplified pre-existing vulnerabilities rather than creating new ones, revealing stress as both acute and chronic in nature.

This chapter then explores the cascading consequences of stress across three interconnected levels: individual professionals, patient care and healthcare organisations. At the individual level, chronic stress is linked to burnout, mental health disorders, compassion fatigue and elevated suicide risk. At the patient level, staff stress and burnout are associated with increased medical errors, reduced quality of care and diminished patient trust. At the organisational level, stress contributes to turnover, financial costs, weakened organisational culture, reduced psychological safety and impaired resilience.

By adopting a systemic perspective, this chapter emphasises the interdependence of these outcomes and challenges reductionist approaches that focus solely on individual resilience. It concludes that sustainable healthcare requires organisational and policy-level interventions that recognise staff well-being as a foundational condition for patient safety, quality of care and long-term system sustainability.

Keywords: Healthcare stress; burnout; high-pressure work environments; patient safety; organisational resilience

1.1 HEALTHCARE AS A HIGH-PRESSURE ENVIRONMENT

Healthcare has long been recognised as one of the most challenging and high-pressure work environments (Riemma et al., 2025). The very nature of healthcare work – where professionals make life-and-death decisions under conditions of uncertainty, limited resources and time constraints – creates an inherent level of stress that distinguishes it from most other occupational contexts (Shanafelt et al., 2015). Unlike many sectors, the costs of errors in healthcare are not simply financial or reputational but can have irreversible consequences for patient safety and public trust (West et al., 2018). This high-stakes character has been described as a defining feature of the healthcare profession, shaping not only the experiences of physicians and nurses but also the organisational cultures in which they operate.

The intensity of the healthcare environment arises from multiple, overlapping sources. On the one hand, there are *structural pressures*, such as understaffing, long shifts and increasingly complex clinical procedures. Studies have repeatedly shown that extended working hours and high patient-to-staff ratios are strongly associated with burnout, fatigue and reduced quality of care (Aiken et al., 2002; Dall'Ora et al., 2015). On the other hand, *emotional and psychological demands* also play a significant role. Healthcare professionals are constantly exposed to human suffering, ethical dilemmas and the need to maintain empathy while preserving professional detachment (D'Avino et al., 2024; Maben et al., 2012). The combination of technical and emotional labour places healthcare workers in what Maslach and Leiter (2016) describe as 'double jeopardy': the simultaneous challenge of managing workload and sustaining emotional engagement.

The COVID-19 pandemic has further magnified these pressures, making them visible to the public in unprecedented ways. Healthcare workers worldwide reported soaring levels of stress, anxiety and depression during the crisis, with systematic reviews confirming a sharp increase in mental health risks (Pappa et al., 2020; Shaukat et al., 2020). The pandemic did not create stress in healthcare but rather exposed and intensified pre-existing structural weaknesses (de Gennaro et al., 2022) – such as chronic understaffing, inadequate protective equipment and insufficient psychosocial support (Kinman et al., 2020). As Greenberg (2020) argues, healthcare during COVID-19 was not only a medical emergency but also a 'psychological hazard,' producing trauma-like experiences for many professionals on the front line.

Another defining feature of healthcare as a high-pressure environment is the *relational complexity* of the work. Healthcare professionals must navigate multiple, often competing, demands: from patients and their families, from colleagues within multidisciplinary teams and from organisational policies and performance targets (Cummings et al., 2018). These intersecting pressures can create role conflict and role ambiguity, which the organisational psychology literature identifies as key predictors of occupational stress (Kahn et al., 1964; Sonnentag & Frese, 2013). For instance, a nurse may face the ethical tension between the time-intensive needs of a critically ill patient and the institutional demand to maintain efficiency across an entire ward. Such dilemmas are not easily resolved and contribute to what has been called the 'moral distress' of healthcare workers (Rushton, 2018).

Moreover, healthcare systems are increasingly affected by *external drivers of pressure*, including demographic shifts, technological innovations and rising patient expectations. Ageing populations have led to higher prevalence of chronic conditions, increasing both the complexity and the volume of care required (World Health Organization, 2016). At the same time, digital health technologies and algorithmic decision-making introduce new opportunities but also new forms of stress, as professionals must adapt to changing workflows and maintain responsibility in the face of technological uncertainty (Büchi et al., 2020; Topol, 2019). These external forces contribute to what Bakker and Demerouti (2017) frame within the Job Demands–Resources (JD-R) model: as demands grow without sufficient resources to meet them, the risk of burnout and disengagement becomes acute.

Importantly, healthcare is not uniformly high-pressure in all contexts; variations exist across specialties, settings and even countries. Emergency departments and intensive care units, for example, are consistently identified as the most stressful environments due to the unpredictability and immediacy of clinical situations (Adriaenssens et al., 2015). Yet even in community and primary care, professionals face unique forms of stress linked to workload, bureaucratic burden and patient complexity (Krasner et al., 2009). Comparative studies have shown that while the intensity and form of stressors may differ, the overarching theme of healthcare as a demanding environment holds across diverse healthcare systems (Lasalvia et al., 2009).

Taken together, these findings portray healthcare as an environment where high pressure is not an exception but a defining feature of daily practice. This recognition is critical not only for academic understanding but also for organisational and policy design. If stress is intrinsic to healthcare, then the challenge is not to eliminate it but to manage it in ways that preserve the well-being of professionals while safeguarding the quality of patient care. As West et al. (2020) emphasise, healthcare organisations that acknowledge and address this dual responsibility – supporting staff while ensuring safety – are more likely to achieve both resilience and sustainability in the long term.

1.2 FROM COVID-19 TO CHRONIC CHALLENGES: WHY STRESS IS NOT A TEMPORARY CRISIS

The COVID-19 pandemic was a watershed moment in the history of healthcare, not because it introduced stress into the sector – stress was already endemic – but because it amplified existing vulnerabilities and made them visible on a global scale (de Gennaro et al., 2022). During the acute phases of the pandemic, healthcare professionals were forced to work under extraordinary conditions: inadequate protective equipment, overwhelming patient loads, ethical dilemmas regarding rationing of care and an unprecedented degree of personal risk (Greenberg et al., 2020; Lai et al., 2020). The magnitude of this experience led to widespread recognition of healthcare workers as being 'at the frontline' not only of the virus but also of a psychological and organisational emergency. Systematic reviews and meta-analyses have documented elevated prevalence of anxiety, depression, post-traumatic stress symptoms and burnout among healthcare workers during COVID-19, with prevalence rates for some conditions exceeding 40% (Pappa et al., 2020; Sanghera et al., 2020).

Yet framing COVID-19-related stress as an exceptional episode risks obscuring a deeper truth: the crisis did not create the fundamental problems of healthcare stress but rather intensified structural challenges that were already present. Long before the pandemic, scholars had documented high rates of burnout among physicians and nurses across different countries and specialties (Maslach & Leiter, 2016; Shanafelt et al., 2012). The causes were remarkably consistent: chronic understaffing, excessive workloads, administrative burdens and the emotional toll of patient care. For example, Aiken et al. (2002) showed that higher nurse-to-patient ratios were directly associated with increased burnout and poorer patient outcomes, a finding that has been replicated in multiple contexts. In this sense, COVID-19 can be seen as a stress test for healthcare systems, revealing how fragile many were even under 'normal' conditions.

A critical insight emerging from the literature is that *stress in healthcare is both acute and chronic.* Acute stressors – such as emergency situations or sudden surges in patient demand – are compounded by chronic stressors, including persistent workforce shortages, limited career progression and organisational cultures that stigmatise vulnerability (West et al., 2018). The pandemic may have generated acute stress of unparalleled intensity, but it also highlighted the chronic conditions of healthcare delivery that ensure stress will remain a permanent challenge unless addressed systemically. As Kinman et al. (2020) argue, healthcare professionals face a 'triple burden' of clinical, emotional and organisational demands that accumulate over time.

The idea that stress in healthcare is not a temporary crisis is further supported by *demographic and systemic trends.* Ageing populations across Europe, North America and parts of Asia are driving an exponential increase in demand for healthcare services (World Health Organization, 2016). At the same time, shortages in the healthcare workforce are projected to worsen, with the WHO estimating a global shortfall of 10 million health workers by 2030 (WHO, 2020). These trends ensure that the mismatch between demands and resources – a central driver of stress in the JD-R model (Bakker & Demerouti, 2017) – will not resolve itself spontaneously. Without targeted interventions, the pandemic's acute crisis will merely transition into an era of sustained and normalised high-pressure work (Riemma et al., 2025).

Moreover, the *bureaucratic and technological landscapes* of healthcare add layers of complexity to this chronic stress. Increasing regulatory requirements and documentation demands consume significant proportions of clinicians' time, often at the expense of patient interaction and professional fulfilment (Shanafelt et al., 2016). While digital health innovations and artificial intelligence promise to alleviate some of these burdens, their implementation can also be a source of stress, requiring new competencies and generating uncertainty about accountability (Del Barone et al., 2025; Gagliarducci & de Gennaro, 2020; Topol, 2019). Thus, the future trajectory of healthcare stress is unlikely to be one of simple relief; rather, it is one of evolving forms of pressure that require adaptive coping and organisational redesign.

Finally, there is growing recognition that *stress in healthcare has ripple effects beyond the individual professional.* Chronic stress and burnout are associated with higher rates of medical error, lower patient satisfaction and increased turnover, creating cycles of strain that further destabilise healthcare systems (Panagioti et al., 2018). In this sense, stress is not only an occupational health issue but also a systemic risk to the quality and sustainability of care. Viewing stress as a temporary crisis underestimates its profound organisational and societal implications. Instead, as West et al. (2020) argue, sustainable healthcare requires acknowledging the centrality of staff well-being as a prerequisite for safe, effective and compassionate patient care.

1.3 CONSEQUENCES FOR PROFESSIONALS, PATIENTS AND ORGANISATIONS

The consequences of stress in healthcare are profound, multifaceted and interdependent. Stress cannot be understood merely as an individual psychological experience; it reverberates through professional well-being, patient safety and outcomes and the performance and sustainability of entire healthcare organisations. This section explores these cascading consequences across three levels of analysis – individual, patient and organisational – emphasising how they are tightly interconnected.

1.3.1 Stress and the Individual Professional

Healthcare professionals face unique occupational hazards when it comes to stress and burnout. Research consistently demonstrates that burnout among physicians and nurses is higher than in many other professions (Rotenstein et al., 2018; Shanafelt et al., 2012). Burnout, classically defined as a syndrome of emotional exhaustion, depersonalisation and reduced personal accomplishment (Maslach & Jackson, 1981), represents both a psychological and physiological toll. Chronic exposure to high job demands is associated with increased risk of depression, anxiety disorders, sleep problems, substance misuse and even suicidal ideation among healthcare workers (Dutheil et al., 2019; West et al., 2016).

A particularly troubling outcome is the elevated suicide risk among physicians and nurses. Studies have found that physicians die by suicide at rates significantly higher than the general population, with female physicians at especially high risk (Schernhammer & Colditz, 2004). Similarly, nurses report high levels of suicidal ideation linked to chronic workplace stressors, bullying and lack of organisational support (Davidson et al., 2020). These findings highlight that stress in healthcare is not merely a matter of reduced job satisfaction or absenteeism (Briganti et al., 2023); it has life-and-death consequences for professionals themselves.

Moreover, stress erodes the intrinsic motivation that drives many to enter healthcare. Professions grounded in altruism and patient care often rely on the emotional commitment of staff. When stress and burnout set in, compassion fatigue can emerge, characterised by emotional numbing, cynicism and a diminished capacity for empathy (Figley, 2002; Peters, 2018). Compassion fatigue is particularly dangerous because it directly undermines the therapeutic relationship between provider and patient, threatening the core mission of healthcare work.

1.3.2 Stress and Patient Care

The consequences of stress among healthcare professionals inevitably extend to patients. Burnout is strongly associated with higher rates of medical error, lower patient satisfaction and diminished quality of care (Panagioti et al., 2018; Tawfik et al., 2019). For example, a systematic review and meta-analysis by Hall et al. (2016) demonstrated that healthcare staff well-being is significantly correlated with patient safety outcomes. Stressed or exhausted professionals are more likely to commit errors in diagnosis, prescribing or procedural execution – errors that can have catastrophic outcomes in high-stakes clinical settings.

Patient experience is also compromised when healthcare providers are stressed. Communication, empathy and trust – central pillars of effective care – are all impaired under conditions of chronic stress (West et al., 2018). Patients perceive when providers are rushed, distracted or emotionally distant, which erodes trust in the healthcare system as a whole. Furthermore, continuity of care suffers when stressed professionals withdraw, reduce working hours or leave the profession altogether, creating instability in patient-provider relationships (Dyrbye et al., 2020).

These issues highlight a vicious cycle: poor patient outcomes increase the moral distress of healthcare professionals, which in turn exacerbates their stress levels (Rushton, 2018). This cycle reveals the systemic nature of stress in healthcare, where harm to patients and harm to professionals are deeply intertwined rather than separate phenomena.

1.3.3 Stress and Organisations

At the organisational level, the impact of stress is equally significant. Burnout and stress contribute to absenteeism, presenteeism, reduced productivity and higher turnover rates (Garcia et al., 2020; Shanafelt et al., 2017). Replacing a single physician who leaves due to burnout has been estimated to cost more than $250,000 when factoring in recruitment, onboarding and lost revenue (Han et al., 2019). For nurses, high turnover destabilises staffing levels and increases workload for remaining staff, perpetuating the cycle of stress and attrition (Dall'Ora et al., 2020).

Financial costs, however, tell only part of the story. Stress also undermines organisational culture. Work environments characterised by high stress often develop cultures of silence, where professionals hesitate to voice concerns for fear of stigma or reprisal (Edmondson, 2019). This erodes psychological safety – a critical factor in promoting learning, error reporting and innovation in healthcare teams. Without psychological safety, organisations risk perpetuating errors and discouraging collective problem-solving, further compromising patient safety and staff well-being.

Moreover, chronic stress and burnout contribute to reputational risks for healthcare organisations. Patient satisfaction scores, quality ratings and public trust are all negatively influenced by the morale and well-being of healthcare staff (Boamah et al., 2018). In an era of increasing transparency and accountability, where outcomes and patient experiences are publicly reported, organisations that fail to address stress risk both regulatory scrutiny and diminished competitiveness.

Stress also undermines the *capacity for organizational resilience* (Del Barone et al., 2025). Healthcare systems frequently face shocks, from pandemics to financial crises, but their ability to adapt depends on the stability and engagement of their workforce (Lengnick-Hall et al., 2011). Burnout weakens this adaptive capacity, leaving organisations less able to respond to crises or to implement innovations such as digital transformation or integrated care pathways (Buonocore et al., 2024). In this sense, stress is not merely a symptom of systemic dysfunction but also a barrier to reform and progress.

1.3.4 A Systemic View: Interdependence of Consequences

While it is analytically useful to separate the consequences of stress into individual, patient and organisational levels, in practice, these levels are deeply interconnected. A physician suffering from burnout may be more likely to make errors, which harms patients and erodes organisational performance metrics. A nurse who leaves due to stress exacerbates staffing shortages, increasing workloads for remaining colleagues and further endangering patient safety. These interdependencies create self-reinforcing cycles of harm that make stress in healthcare a systemic challenge rather than an individual failing (West et al., 2020).

For this reason, interventions that target only one level of consequence – for example, resilience training for individuals without addressing organisational drivers – are unlikely to succeed in the long term. Sustainable solutions require integrated approaches that recognise the cascading effects of stress across the professional, patient and organisational domains.

REFERENCES

Adriaenssens, J., De Gucht, V., & Maes, S. (2015). Determinants and prevalence of burnout in emergency nurses: A systematic review of 25 years of research. *International Journal of Nursing Studies*, *52*(2), 649–661.

Aiken, L. H., Clarke, S. P., Sloane, D. M., Sochalski, J., & Silber, J. H. (2002). Hospital nurse staffing and patient mortality, nurse burnout, and job dissatisfaction. *JAMA*, *288*(16), 1987–1993.

Bakker, A. B., & Demerouti, E. (2017). Job demands–resources theory: Taking stock and looking forward. *Journal of Occupational Health Psychology*, *22*(3), 273–285.

Boamah, S. A., Spence Laschinger, H. K., Wong, C., & Clarke, S. (2018). Effect of transformational leadership on job satisfaction and patient safety outcomes. *Nursing Outlook*, *66*(2), 180–189.

Briganti, P., de Gennaro, D., Buonocore, F., & Varriale, L. (2023). Job (dis-) satisfaction in pay-for-performance health care contexts: A meta-synthesis of qualitative literature. *International Journal of Public Sector Management*, *36*(6/7), 606–631. https://doi.org/10.1108/IJPSM-02-2023-0061

Büchi, M., Festic, N., & Latzer, M. (2020). Digital overuse and subjective well-being in a digitized society. *Social Indicators Research*, *150*(2), 591–613.

Buonocore, F., Annosi, M. C., de Gennaro, D., & Riemma, F. (2024). Digital transformation and social change: Leadership strategies for responsible innovation. *Journal of Engineering and Technology Management*, *74*, 1–14. https://doi.org/10.1016/j.jengtecman.2024.101843

Cummings, G. G., Tate, K., Lee, S., Wong, C. A., Paananen, T., Micaroni, S. P., & Chatterjee, G. E. (2018). Leadership styles and outcome patterns for the nursing workforce and work environment: A systematic review. *International Journal of Nursing Studies*, *85*, 19–60.

Dall'Ora, C., Ball, J., Reinius, M., & Griffiths, P. (2020). Burnout in nursing: A theoretical review. *Human Resources for Health*, *18*(1), 41.

Dall'Ora, C., Griffiths, P., Ball, J., Simon, M., & Aiken, L. H. (2015). Association of 12 h shifts and nurses' job satisfaction, burnout and intention to leave: Findings from a cross-sectional study of 12 European countries. *BMJ Open*, *5*(9), e008331.

Davidson, J. E., Proudfoot, J., Lee, K., Zisook, S., & Newman-Toker, D. (2020). A longitudinal analysis of nurse suicide in the United States (2005–2016). *Archives of Psychiatric Nursing*, *34*(5), 369–376.

D'Avino, E., de Gennaro, D., Inno, L., & Vicentini, G. (2024). Promoting equality through ethical AI and DEI principles: A case study of the LSST. In D. de Gennaro & M. Marino (Eds.), *Global classroom: Multicultural approaches and organizational strategies in teaching and learning business and economics* (pp. 161–166). Emerald Publishing Limited. ISBN: 978-1-83549-285-7. https://doi.org/10.1108/978-1-83549-284-020241020

de Gennaro, D., Loia, F., & Piscopo, G. (2022). Working role of women in a pandemic world: A poetic inquiry. *Management Research Review*, *45*(11), 1373–1392. ISSN: 2040-8269. https://doi.org/10.1108/MRR-06-2021-0430

Del Barone, L., de Gennaro, D., & Buonocore, F. (2025). AI-driven HRM and managerial competencies: Strengthening organizational resilience in public administration. *Management Decision. ahead-of-print*. https://doi.org/10.1108/MD-06-2024-1252

Dutheil, F., Aubert, C., Pereira, B., Dambrun, M., Moustafa, F., Mermillod, M., Baker, J. S., Trousselard, M., Lesage, F. X., & Navel, V. (2019). Suicide among physicians and health-care workers: A systematic review and meta-analysis. *PLoS One*, *14*(12), e0226361.

Dyrbye, L. N., West, C. P., Sinsky, C. A., Goeders, L. E., Satele, D. V., Tutty, M. A., & Shanafelt, T. D. (2020). Medical licensure questions and physician reluctance to seek care for mental health conditions. *Mayo Clinic Proceedings*, *92*(10), 1486–1493.

Edmondson, A. C. (2019). *The fearless organization: Creating psychological safety in the workplace for learning, innovation, and growth*. Wiley.

Figley, C. R. (2002). *Compassion fatigue: Psychotherapists' chronic lack of self care*. Brunner-Routledge.

Gagliarducci, F., & de Gennaro, D. (2020). *A project for assessing public management competencies*. In M. Decastri, S. Battini, F. Buonocore, & F. Gagliarducci (Eds.), *Organizational development in public administration: The Italian way* (pp. 177–212). Palgrave MacMillan. ISBN: 978-30-30437-98-5. https://doi.org/10.1007/978-3-030-43799-2_6

Garcia, C. L., Abreu, L. C., Ramos, J. L., Castro, C. F. D., Smiderle, F. R. N., Santos, J. A. D., & Bezerra, I. M. P. (2020). Influence of burnout on patient safety: Systematic review and meta-analysis. *Medicina*, *56*(12), 737.

Greenberg, N. (2020). Mental health of health-care workers in the COVID-19 era. *Nature Reviews Nephrology*, *16*(8), 425–426.

Greenberg, N., Docherty, M., Gnanapragasam, S., & Wessely, S. (2020). Managing mental health challenges faced by healthcare workers during COVID-19. *BMJ*, *368*, m1211.

Hall, L. H., Johnson, J., Watt, I., Tsipa, A., & O'Connor, D. B. (2016). Healthcare staff well-being, burnout, and patient safety: A systematic review. *PLoS One*, *11*(7), e0159015.

Han, S., Shanafelt, T. D., Sinsky, C. A., Awad, K. M., Dyrbye, L. N., Fiscus, L. C., Trockel, M., & Goh, J. (2019). Estimating the attributable cost of physician burnout in the United States. *Annals of Internal Medicine*, *170* (11), 784–790.

Kahn, R. L., Wolfe, D. M., Quinn, R. P., Snoek, J. D., & Rosenthal, R. A. (1964). *Organizational stress: Studies in role conflict and ambiguity*. Wiley.

Kinman, G., Teoh, K., & Harriss, A. (2020). Supporting the well-being of healthcare workers during and after COVID-19. *Occupational Medicine*, *70* (5), 294–296.

Krasner, M. S., Epstein, R. M., Beckman, H., Suchman, A. L., Chapman, B., Mooney, C. J., & Quill, T. E. (2009). Association of an educational program in mindful communication with burnout, empathy, and attitudes among primary care physicians. *JAMA*, *302*(12), 1284–1293.

Lai, J., Ma, S., Wang, Y., Cai, Z., Hu, J., Wei, N., Wu, J., Du, H., Chen, T., Li, R., Tan, H., Kang, L., Yao, L., Huang, M., Wang, H., Wang, G., Liu, Z., & Hu, S. (2020). Factors associated with mental health outcomes among health care workers exposed to coronavirus disease 2019. *JAMA Network Open*, *3*(3), e203976.

Lasalvia, A., Bonetto, C., Bertani, M., Bissoli, S., Cristofalo, D., Marrella, G., Ceccato, E., Cremonese, C., De Rossi, M., Lazzarotto, L., Marangon, V., Morandi, S., Zucchetto, M., & Ruggeri, M. (2009). Influence of perceived organisational factors on job burnout: Survey of community mental health staff. *British Journal of Psychiatry*, *195*(6), 537–544.

Lengnick-Hall, C. A., Beck, T. E., & Lengnick-Hall, M. L. (2011). Developing a capacity for organizational resilience through strategic human resource management. *Human Resource Management Review*, *21*(3), 243–255.

Maben, J., Adams, M., Peccei, R., Murrells, T., & Robert, G. (2012). 'Poppets and parcels': The links between staff experience of work and acutely ill older peoples' experience of hospital care. *International Journal of Nursing Studies*, *49*(8), 1007–1018.

Maslach, C., & Jackson, S. E. (1981). The measurement of experienced burnout. *Journal of Occupational Behavior*, *2*(2), 99–113.

Maslach, C., & Leiter, M. P. (2016). Burnout: A multidimensional perspective. In C. L. Cooper (Ed.), *The handbook of stress and health* (pp. 34–56). Wiley.

Panagioti, M., Geraghty, K., Johnson, J., Zhou, A., Panagopoulou, E., Chew-Graham, C., Peters, D., Hodkinson, A., Riley, R., & Esmail, A. (2018). Association between physician burnout and patient safety, professionalism, and patient satisfaction: A systematic review and meta-analysis. *JAMA Internal Medicine*, *178*(10), 1317–1330.

Pappa, S., Ntella, V., Giannakas, T., Giannakoulis, V. G., Papoutsi, E., & Katsaounou, P. (2020). Prevalence of depression, anxiety, and insomnia among healthcare workers during the COVID-19 pandemic: A systematic review and meta-analysis. *Brain, Behavior, and Immunity*, *88*, 901–907.

Peters, E. (2018). Compassion fatigue in nursing: A concept analysis. *Nursing Forum*, *53*(4), 466–480.

Riemma, F., Buonocore, F., & de Gennaro, D. (2025). Coping with pressure: Stress management and organizational support in healthcare settings. *Personnel Review. ahead-of-print.* https://doi.org/10.1108/PR-04-2025-0387

Rotenstein, L. S., Torre, M., Ramos, M. A., Rosales, R. C., Guille, C., Sen, S., & Mata, D. A. (2018). Prevalence of burnout among physicians: A systematic review. *JAMA, 320*(11), 1131–1150.

Rushton, C. H. (2018). *Moral resilience: Transforming moral suffering in healthcare*. Oxford University Press.

Sanghera, J., Pattani, N., Hashmi, Y., Varley, K. F., Cheruvu, M. S., Bradley, A., & Burke, J. R. (2020). The impact of SARS-CoV-2 on the mental health of healthcare workers in a hospital setting—A systematic review. *Journal of Occupational Health*, *62*(1), e12175.

Schernhammer, E. S., & Colditz, G. A. (2004). Suicide rates among physicians: A quantitative and gender assessment (meta-analysis). *American Journal of Psychiatry*, *161*(12), 2295–2302.

Shanafelt, T. D., Boone, S., Tan, L., Dyrbye, L. N., Sotile, W., Satele, D., West, C. P., Sloan, J., & Oreskovich, M. R. (2012). Burnout and satisfaction with work-life balance among US physicians relative to the general US population. *Archives of Internal Medicine*, *172*(18), 1377–1385.

Shanafelt, T. D., Dyrbye, L. N., & West, C. P. (2016). Addressing physician burnout: The way forward. *JAMA*, *317*(9), 901–902.

Shanafelt, T. D., Goh, J., & Sinsky, C. (2017). The business case for investing in physician well-being. *JAMA Internal Medicine*, *177*(12), 1826–1832.

Shanafelt, T. D., Hasan, O., Dyrbye, L. N., Sinsky, C., Satele, D., Sloan, J., & West, C. P. (2015). Changes in burnout and satisfaction with work-life balance in physicians and the general US working population between 2011 and 2014. *Mayo Clinic Proceedings*, *90*(12), 1600–1613.

Shaukat, N., Ali, D. M., & Razzak, J. (2020). Physical and mental health impacts of COVID-19 on healthcare workers: A scoping review. *International Journal of Emergency Medicine*, *13*(1), 40.

Sonnentag, S., & Frese, M. (2013). Stress in organizations. In N. W. Schmitt & S. Highhouse (Eds.), *Handbook of psychology: Vol. 12. Industrial and organizational psychology* (2nd ed., pp. 560–592). Wiley.

Tawfik, D. S., Profit, J., Morgenthaler, T. I., Satele, D. V., Sinsky, C. A., Dyrbye, L. N., Tutty, M. A., West, C. P., & Shanafelt, T. D. (2019). Physician burnout, well-being, and work unit safety grades in relationship to reported medical errors. *Mayo Clinic Proceedings*, *93*(11), 1571–1580.

Topol, E. (2019). *Deep medicine: How artificial intelligence can make healthcare human again*. Basic Books.

West, M., Bailey, S., & Williams, E. (2020). *The courage of compassion: Supporting nurses and midwives to deliver high-quality care*. The King's Fund Report.

West, C. P., Dyrbye, L. N., Erwin, P. J., & Shanafelt, T. D. (2018). Interventions to prevent and reduce physician burnout: A systematic review and meta-analysis. *The Lancet*, *388*(10057), 2272–2281.

West, C. P., Dyrbye, L. N., & Shanafelt, T. D. (2016). Physician burnout: Contributors, consequences, and solutions. *Journal of Internal Medicine*, *283*(6), 516–529.

World Health Organization. (2016). *Global strategy on human resources for health: Workforce 2030*. WHO.

World Health Organization. (2020). *State of the World's nursing 2020: Investing in education, jobs and leadership*. WHO.

2

MAPPING THE TERRAIN: THEORIES OF STRESS AND COPING

ABSTRACT

This chapter maps the principal theoretical frameworks used to understand stress and coping in healthcare, highlighting their relevance, complementarities and limitations in high-demand clinical contexts. It first examines the Transactional Model of Stress and Coping, emphasising the role of cognitive appraisal, meaning-making and coping strategies in shaping healthcare professionals' stress experiences. This chapter illustrates how problem-focused and emotion-focused coping operate in healthcare practice and underscores the importance of situational fit and moral appraisal, particularly in ethically demanding environments.

This chapter then reviews two structural models of occupational stress: the Demand–Control model and the Effort–Reward Imbalance model. These frameworks shift attention from individual appraisal to organisational conditions, demonstrating how limited autonomy, insufficient social support, lack of recognition and overcommitment contribute to chronic stress and burnout among healthcare workers. Empirical evidence from diverse healthcare settings confirms the explanatory power of these models in predicting burnout, job dissatisfaction and turnover intentions.

Building on these foundations, this chapter introduces the Job Demands–Resources (JD-R) framework as an integrative and dynamic model particularly suited to healthcare. The JD-R model captures both health impairment and motivational processes and explicitly incorporates resilience as a key personal and organisational resource. Finally, the chapter explores proactive approaches such as job crafting and playful work design, highlighting how healthcare professionals can actively reshape tasks, relationships and cognitive frames to buffer stress and sustain engagement. This chapter concludes that contemporary stress theory in healthcare must integrate individual, collective and organisational perspectives to support sustainable well-being and performance.

Keywords: Stress and coping theories; transactional model; Job Demands–Resources framework; resilience; job crafting

2.1 THE TRANSACTIONAL MODEL OF STRESS AND COPING IN HEALTHCARE PRACTICE

The Transactional Model of Stress and Coping, first articulated by Lazarus and Folkman (1984), remains one of the most influential frameworks for understanding how individuals experience and respond to stress. The model conceptualises stress not as a direct stimulus or response but as a dynamic transaction between the individual and their environment, mediated by cognitive appraisal and coping strategies (Buonocore et al., 2020). This perspective is particularly well-suited to healthcare, where stress emerges from the continuous negotiation between professional demands, available resources and individual meaning-making processes.

At its core, the model posits that stress occurs when individuals appraise situations as taxing or exceeding their resources and endangering their well-being. Primary appraisal involves evaluating whether an event is irrelevant, benign-positive or stressful; if stressful, it may be appraised as a harm/loss, a threat or a challenge (Lazarus & Folkman, 1984). In healthcare practice, such appraisals are omnipresent. For example, a nurse confronted with an acutely deteriorating patient may appraise the situation as a threat if resources are insufficient, as a harm/loss if the outcome seems inevitable, or as a challenge if they feel confident in their clinical skills and team support (Folkman et al., 1986).

Secondary appraisal refers to the evaluation of coping resources and options. Healthcare professionals engage in constant assessments of whether they have the knowledge, time, institutional support and personal resilience to respond effectively. For instance, studies of intensive care unit (ICU) nurses show that their stress levels are moderated not only by patient acuity but also by their perceived ability to access team collaboration and institutional backing (Poncet et al., 2007). Thus, the transactional perspective highlights the subjective and context-dependent nature of stress in healthcare: the same clinical event can produce widely divergent stress experiences depending on appraisal processes and available coping mechanisms.

Coping, in this model, is defined as the constantly changing cognitive and behavioural efforts to manage specific external and/or internal demands appraised as taxing or exceeding one's resources (Lazarus & Folkman, 1984). Coping strategies are typically divided into problem-focused and emotion-focused approaches. Problem-focused coping involves efforts to address the source of stress directly, such as seeking information, reorganising work tasks or advocating for additional resources. Emotion-focused coping, by contrast, involves attempts to regulate emotional responses, such as using humour, detachment or social support (Carver et al., 1989).

In healthcare, both types of coping are evident, and their balance depends heavily on context. For example, physicians facing diagnostic uncertainty may employ problem-focused coping by consulting guidelines or colleagues, whereas nurses dealing with the death of a patient may rely on emotion-focused coping to manage grief (Healy & McKay, 2000). Importantly, neither strategy is inherently adaptive nor maladaptive; their effectiveness depends on the match between coping efforts and situational demands (Lazarus, 1999). This principle, known as the 'goodness-of-fit' hypothesis, has been empirically supported in healthcare contexts. For instance, problem-focused coping is more effective in controllable situations, while emotion-focused coping may be more beneficial when stressors are uncontrollable, such as terminal illness or patient death (Folkman & Moskowitz, 2004).

Several empirical studies have applied the transactional model to healthcare workers. A seminal study by Tyler and Cushway (1995) found that nurses' stress levels were strongly predicted by their appraisals of role conflict and lack of control, as well as by their reliance on emotion-focused coping strategies such as avoidance. Similarly, McGrath et al. (2003) reported that junior doctors who engaged in problem-focused coping experienced lower levels of anxiety and higher job satisfaction compared to those who relied primarily on avoidance strategies. More recently, studies in the wake of the COVID-19 pandemic have confirmed that appraisal and coping processes are central to healthcare workers' resilience (Briganti et al., 2023). For example, Huang et al. (2020) found that Chinese nurses who engaged in positive reappraisal and active problem-solving reported lower psychological distress during the pandemic, highlighting the protective role of adaptive coping.

The transactional model also underscores the role of meaning-making in coping. Lazarus (1999) argued that reappraisal processes – where individuals reinterpret stressful events to find positive meaning – are a vital component of resilience. In healthcare, meaning-making is often grounded in professional identity and commitment to patient care. Qualitative research suggests that many healthcare workers frame their struggles within a narrative of vocation and service, which helps sustain them in the face of adversity (Rushton, 2018). However, when institutional values conflict with personal values – such as when cost-cutting undermines patient care – moral distress arises, leading to heightened stress and burnout (Epstein & Hamric, 2009).

While the Transactional Model provides a powerful lens, scholars have noted some limitations when applied to healthcare. First, the model's emphasis on individual appraisal risks underestimating the role of organisational and systemic factors. For example, secondary appraisal of coping resources is not purely individual but deeply shaped by staffing policies, leadership practices and institutional culture (LeBlanc, 2009). Second, the model pays less attention to collective coping strategies, which are increasingly recognised as crucial in healthcare teams (Slišković, 2017). These limitations suggest the need to expand the model to incorporate organisational and collective dimensions – a point that later chapters of this book will address.

Nevertheless, the Transactional Model remains a cornerstone in understanding stress and coping in healthcare. It highlights the subjective nature of stress, the centrality of appraisal processes and the adaptive potential of coping strategies. By applying this framework, researchers and practitioners can better appreciate the variability in stress responses among healthcare professionals and design interventions that enhance adaptive coping while addressing the structural factors that constrain it (e.g., Buonocore et al., 2021).

2.2 DEMAND–CONTROL AND EFFORT–REWARD: THE ROLE OF RESOURCES AND RECOGNITION

Two of the most influential models for understanding occupational stress, particularly in healthcare, are Karasek's Demand–Control model (Karasek, 1979; Karasek & Theorell, 1990) and Siegrist's Effort–Reward Imbalance (ERI) model (Siegrist, 1996). Together, these frameworks emphasise the interplay between job demands, the degree of autonomy and control available to workers and the balance between the efforts expended and the rewards received. Both models have been extensively applied in healthcare research, yielding insights into how structural and organisational factors shape stress, burnout and professional well-being.

2.2.1 The Demand–Control Model in Healthcare

The Demand–Control model proposes that occupational stress results from the interaction of two primary factors: job demands (e.g., workload, time pressure, role conflict) and job control (the degree of autonomy in decision-making and skill use). Jobs characterised by high demands and low control – so-called 'high-strain jobs' – are the most likely to produce stress and adverse health outcomes (Karasek, 1979; Riemma et al., 2025).

Healthcare settings often epitomise this high-strain profile. Nurses and physicians face immense cognitive and emotional demands, often coupled with rigid organisational structures that limit their autonomy (Theorell & Karasek, 1996). For example, research has shown that nurses working in acute care units frequently report high patient loads, conflicting role expectations and little influence over staffing decisions, creating conditions consistent with high-strain jobs (Van der Doef & Maes, 1999). Physicians similarly encounter high demands in terms of clinical workload and administrative tasks, while feeling constrained by bureaucratic procedures and limited control over resource allocation (Linzer et al., 2000).

Empirical evidence supports the predictive power of the Demand–Control model in healthcare. Bourbonnais et al. (1999) found that nurses exposed to high psychological demands and low decision latitude had a significantly higher risk of burnout and psychological distress. Likewise, studies of physicians confirm that limited autonomy – particularly when combined with high time pressure – predicts higher levels of job dissatisfaction and intention to leave the profession (Shanafelt et al., 2009).

Interestingly, Karasek's model also incorporates the concept of social support, later expanded into the 'Demand–Control–Support' model. In healthcare, support from colleagues and supervisors can buffer the effects of high demands, mitigating stress and protecting against burnout (de Jonge et al., 2000). For instance, studies of ICUs demonstrate that supportive team environments can reduce the adverse impact of high patient acuity and long shifts on staff well-being (Poncet et al., 2007). This underscores the collective nature of stress experiences in healthcare: autonomy and support are not solely individual resources but embedded in team and organisational structures.

2.2.2 The ERI Model in Healthcare

While the Demand–Control model emphasises job characteristics, Siegrist's ERI model focuses on the social reciprocity inherent in the employment relationship (see Annosi et al., 2025). According to this framework, stress arises when high effort at work is not met with commensurate rewards in terms of salary, esteem or career opportunities (Siegrist, 1996). Healthcare is particularly prone to such imbalances, as professionals often invest extraordinary effort – long hours, emotional labour and personal sacrifice – without adequate recognition or reward.

Several studies have validated the ERI model in healthcare contexts. Peter et al. (1998) found that German hospital workers experiencing ERI had higher risks of cardiovascular disease, confirming the model's physiological relevance. Li et al. (2014) reported that Chinese nurses exposed to high ERI had significantly greater odds of depressive symptoms and burnout. In a large European study, Mark and Smith (2012) showed that healthcare employees perceiving high ERI also reported higher intentions to quit and lower organisational commitment.

Importantly, the ERI model also accounts for overcommitment, defined as a motivational pattern characterised by excessive striving and inability to withdraw from work. Healthcare professionals frequently exhibit overcommitment due to vocational identity and professional ethos (Siegrist, 1996; van Vegchel et al., 2005). While overcommitment may initially appear adaptive, enabling professionals to meet extreme demands, it eventually exacerbates strain and increases vulnerability to burnout. For example, a longitudinal study by Bakker et al. (2000) showed that Dutch nurses with high overcommitment and ERI reported significantly higher levels of emotional exhaustion.

2.2.3 Integrating the Two Models: Resources and Recognition

Although conceptually distinct, the Demand–Control and ERI models converge on a central insight: resources and recognition are critical in shaping stress outcomes. Autonomy and social support (from the Demand–Control model) and esteem and fairness (from the ERI model) both act as protective resources that buffer the negative effects of high demands. When these resources are absent, stress becomes chronic and corrosive.

In practice, healthcare organisations often fail to provide sufficient resources or recognition. Chronic understaffing and rigid hierarchies reduce autonomy, while inadequate pay, limited promotion opportunities and lack of appreciation contribute to ERI (Briganti et al., 2023; Laschinger & Finegan, 2005). Moreover, the cultural expectation that healthcare workers should be altruistically motivated can normalise imbalances, making professionals reluctant to demand recognition (Grace & VanHeuvelen, 2019).

Integrating these models with the broader Job Demands–Resources (JD-R) framework suggests that interventions must simultaneously address structural resources (autonomy, staffing, support) and social reciprocity (fair pay, recognition, career development). Evidence indicates that organisations investing in supportive leadership, participatory decision-making and recognition programs see measurable improvements in both staff well-being and patient outcomes (Cummings et al., 2018; Shanafelt & Noseworthy, 2017).

2.3 TOWARDS UPDATED MODELS: RESILIENCE AND THE JD-R FRAMEWORK

While the Transactional Model of Stress and Coping (Lazarus & Folkman, 1984), the Demand–Control model (Karasek, 1979; Karasek & Theorell, 1990), and the ERI model (Siegrist, 1996) remain foundational, the complexity of healthcare work has spurred scholars to adopt more integrative frameworks. Among these, the JD-R model (Demerouti et al., 2001; Bakker & Demerouti, 2007) has become one of the most influential in recent decades. The JD-R framework not only captures the role of demands and resources but also integrates the concept of resilience, offering a dynamic and flexible model well-suited to healthcare environments.

2.3.1 The JD-R Model: Core Assumptions

The JD-R model posits that every occupation has its own specific risk factors associated with job stress, which can be categorised into job demands and job resources (Demerouti et al., 2001).

- Job demands refer to aspects of the job that require sustained effort and are associated with physiological or psychological costs, such as workload, emotional demands and time pressure.
- Job resources, in contrast, are aspects that help achieve work goals, reduce job demands or stimulate personal growth, including autonomy, feedback, support and recognition.

Crucially, the JD-R model proposes two psychological processes:

(1) A health impairment process, where excessive demands deplete energy and lead to burnout.

(2) A motivational process, where resources foster engagement, resilience and performance.

In healthcare, these dual processes are clearly visible. For instance, high patient loads and constant exposure to suffering contribute to exhaustion (Aiken et al., 2002; Dall'Ora et al., 2015), while supportive leadership, teamwork and recognition buffer these effects and enhance engagement (Cummings et al., 2018; Shanafelt & Noseworthy, 2017).

2.3.2 Resilience as a Key Mediator

A major advance in the application of the JD-R model to healthcare has been the integration of resilience – both individual and organisational – as a mediating and moderating construct. Resilience is typically defined as the ability to adapt positively in the face of adversity, maintaining or regaining well-being and performance (Fletcher & Sarkar, 2013).

At the individual level, resilience enables healthcare professionals to cope with high demands without succumbing to burnout. Studies show that resilient nurses and physicians are more likely to engage in adaptive coping strategies, sustain empathy and recover more quickly from stressful events (Mealer et al., 2012; Hart et al., 2014). For example, a study of ICU nurses demonstrated that resilience mediated the relationship between emotional demands and psychological distress, suggesting that resilience functions as a protective personal resource (Mealer et al., 2012).

At the organisational level, resilience refers to the capacity of healthcare systems to adapt and continue functioning under stress, such as during pandemics or resource shortages (Lengnick-Hall et al., 2011). The COVID-19 pandemic underscored that organisational resilience – through flexible staffing, clear communication and visible leadership – was critical in sustaining care delivery and staff morale (de Gennaro et al., 2022; Maunder et al., 2021; Shaukat et al., 2020).

The JD-R model thus provides a framework for integrating resilience into stress theory: resilience is both a personal resource that mitigates the health impairment process and a driver of the motivational process that enhances engagement.

2.3.3 Evidence From Healthcare Research

Empirical studies have applied the JD-R model to diverse healthcare settings, consistently confirming its explanatory power. Bakker et al. (2004) found that job demands predicted exhaustion among healthcare workers, while job resources predicted engagement, with both processes independently affecting performance. Similarly, Van Bogaert et al. (2013) demonstrated that supportive nurse practice environments (resources) reduced burnout and improved job satisfaction, even in the context of high demands.

Recent studies during the COVID-19 pandemic further highlight the JD-R framework's relevance. Zhang et al. (2021) found that frontline nurses with higher perceived resources – such as team support and organisational recognition – reported lower burnout and higher resilience, despite extreme demands. Another study by Serrano-Ripoll et al. (2020) showed that interventions providing psychological support and resources significantly reduced mental health risks among healthcare workers, aligning with the JD-R prediction that resources buffer the impact of demands.

2.3.4 Extending the JD-R Framework

The JD-R model's flexibility allows for the integration of personal resources – such as optimism, self-efficacy and resilience – into the model (Xanthopoulou et al., 2007). This is particularly valuable in healthcare, where individual differences strongly influence stress and coping outcomes. For example, Schwarzer and Hallum (2008) demonstrated that self-efficacy moderated the relationship between job stress and burnout among teachers, a finding echoed in healthcare contexts with resilience (Hart et al., 2014).

Additionally, scholars are increasingly recognising the importance of collective resources, such as team cohesion and psychological safety. These collective dimensions extend the JD-R model beyond the individual, acknowledging that healthcare is fundamentally a team-based endeavour (Edmondson, 2019). Teams with high psychological safety and shared resilience are better able to adapt to stressors, avoid errors and maintain morale (West et al., 2020).

2.4 JOB CRAFTING AND PLAYFUL WORK DESIGN (PWD) AS RESOURCES AGAINST STRESS AND BURNOUT[1]

In recent years, the literature on occupational stress and well-being has increasingly moved beyond deficit-based perspectives to explore proactive strategies that individuals can use to reshape their work experiences (Tomo & de Gennaro, 2020). Among the most influential concepts emerging from this shift are job crafting (Wrzesniewski & Dutton, 2001) and the more recent idea of PWD (Petrou et al., 2012; Tims et al., 2013; van Wingerden & Poell, 2019). Both approaches emphasise the agency of employees in shaping their tasks, relationships and cognitive frames in ways that reduce stress and enhance engagement. Within healthcare – a sector characterised by high demands, frequent exposure to suffering and organisational constraints – such proactive strategies may be particularly critical in buffering against burnout and supporting resilience.

2.4.1 The Concept of Job Crafting

Job crafting refers to the self-initiated changes that employees make to their job tasks, relationships and perceptions in order to better align work with their strengths, values and needs (Wrzesniewski & Dutton, 2001). Three main dimensions have been identified: task crafting (altering the type, scope or number of tasks), relational crafting (changing the nature or extent of interactions with others) and cognitive crafting (reframing the meaning or purpose of work) (de Gennaro, 2019; Lazazzara et al., 2020). Later operationalisations within the JD-R framework have highlighted two broad categories of job crafting behaviours: increasing structural and social resources (e.g., seeking feedback, learning opportunities, supportive relationships) and increasing challenging demands (e.g., proactively taking on projects that foster growth) while decreasing hindering demands (e.g., reducing emotionally draining tasks) (Demerouti, 2014; Tims et al., 2012).

The potential of job crafting to mitigate stress and burnout is grounded in several mechanisms. By proactively adjusting tasks or relationships, employees can restore a better person–job fit (Kristof-Brown et al., 2005), thereby reducing the strain associated with misalignment. Cognitive crafting, in particular, enables professionals to reconnect with the meaningful aspects of their work, which research shows is a strong buffer against emotional exhaustion (Berg et al., 2013). Importantly, job crafting is not only an individual coping strategy (e.g., Buonocore et al., 2022) but also a way of shaping the psychosocial environment, fostering greater autonomy, support and resource availability – all of which are known predictors of reduced burnout (Bakker & Demerouti, 2017).

2.4.2 Job Crafting in Healthcare

Healthcare provides a fertile ground for examining job crafting because of its dual characteristics: high demands and high potential for meaningfulness. Studies show that nurses, physicians and allied health professionals frequently engage in job crafting, particularly relational and cognitive forms. For instance, nurses often reframe routine tasks, such as administering medication, as opportunities to connect with patients, thereby imbuing technical duties with relational significance (Leana et al., 2009). Physicians facing bureaucratic overload may engage in cognitive crafting by emphasising the life-saving aspects of their role, which helps sustain motivation under pressure (Riemma et al., 2025; Vogt et al., 2016).

Empirical research supports the protective effects of job crafting in healthcare. Rudolph et al. (2017) found that healthcare workers who engaged in job crafting reported lower levels of burnout and higher levels of engagement, even under high demand conditions. van Wingerden et al. (2017) demonstrated in an intervention study that job crafting training improved nurses' resource-seeking behaviours and reduced emotional exhaustion. Petrou et al. (2012) showed that employees who actively increased job resources during organisational change experienced less strain and more work engagement. These findings suggest that job crafting functions as a proactive coping mechanism, enabling healthcare professionals to counterbalance stressors by mobilising and creating resources.

2.4.3 Playful Work Design

Building on the insights of job crafting, scholars have recently proposed the notion of PWD as another avenue for mitigating stress and enhancing resilience. PWD refers to employees' ability to proactively introduce elements of play, fun and challenge into their work, thereby transforming demanding or monotonous tasks into more intrinsically motivating experiences (Bakker et al., 2008; Petrou et al., 2015). Unlike traditional job crafting, which often emphasises structural changes or cognitive reframing (see Buonocore et al., 2020), PWD explicitly leverages playfulness as a psychological resource.

The mechanisms of PWD are closely tied to theories of intrinsic motivation and positive psychology (Csikszentmihalyi, 1990). By reframing tasks as challenges or games, employees can enter states of flow, characterised by deep engagement, absorption and enjoyment. Such states not only buffer against stress but also replenish energy and foster creativity (Buonocore et al., 2021; Salanova et al., 2006). For example, a nurse may introduce playful competition into routine administrative tasks to make them more engaging, or a surgical team may develop rituals and humour to maintain morale during long shifts. While PWD has received less empirical attention than job crafting, early studies suggest that it predicts higher engagement, greater resilience and lower exhaustion (Petrou et al., 2015; van Wingerden & Poell, 2019).

2.4.4 Integrating Job Crafting and PWD

Both job crafting and PWD share a common premise: employees are not passive recipients of job demands but active shapers of their work environment. They complement traditional stress theories by emphasising the agency and creativity of professionals in coping with demands. Importantly, these strategies do not deny systemic stressors but provide ways of sustaining energy and meaning within them. In healthcare, where structural constraints are often difficult to eliminate, the ability to craft or playfully redesign work can make the difference between chronic burnout and sustained resilience.

At the same time, both job crafting and PWD are not substitutes for organisational responsibility. They are most effective when supported by cultures that encourage autonomy, psychological safety and innovation (Edmondson, 2019). Without supportive leadership and adequate resources, employees' attempts to craft or playfully redesign their work may be stifled or even punished. For example, a nurse who tries to alter task boundaries to spend more time with patients may be reprimanded in organisations with rigid role definitions. This highlights that proactive strategies thrive in environments where organisational and individual agency converge.

2.4.5 Future Directions

The literature suggests several promising directions for integrating job crafting and PWD into stress management strategies. Interventions that train healthcare workers in job crafting behaviours have already shown effectiveness (Van Wingerden et al., 2017). Future programmes might also incorporate PWD elements, teaching professionals to infuse tasks with fun and creativity as part of resilience training (de Gennaro & Marino, 2024). Research could further explore how PWD interacts with emotional labour and moral distress – two central stressors in healthcare – to determine whether play provides a unique buffer in emotionally demanding contexts.

Additionally, there is scope for investigating how job crafting and PWD operate collectively within teams. Collective job crafting, where groups jointly reshape tasks and interactions, may be particularly relevant in healthcare, where teamwork is central to care delivery (Leana et al., 2009). Playful rituals and shared humour may also reinforce team cohesion, further buffering against stress (Mesmer-Magnus et al., 2012). Such team-level dynamics expand our understanding of resilience from an individual trait to a collective process embedded in social relationships and organisational culture.

NOTE

1. Written by: Filomena Buonocore, Davide de Gennaro, Ludovica Del Barone and Viviana Colombi Evangelista.

REFERENCES

Aiken, L. H., Clarke, S. P., Sloane, D. M., Sochalski, J., & Silber, J. H. (2002). Hospital nurse staffing and patient mortality, nurse burnout, and job dissatisfaction. *JAMA*, *288*(16), 1987–1993.

Annosi, M. C., van der Heijden, B. I. J. M., Karamanavi, D., & de Gennaro, D. (2025). Mutual gains through sustainable employability investments: Integrating HRM practices for organisational competitiveness. *Personnel Review*. https://doi.org/10.1108/PR-05-2024-0515

Bakker, A. B., & Demerouti, E. (2007). The Job Demands–Resources model: State of the art. *Journal of Managerial Psychology*, *22*(3), 309–328.

Bakker, A. B., & Demerouti, E. (2017). Job Demands–Resources theory: Taking stock and looking forward. *Journal of Occupational Health Psychology*, *22*(3), 273–285.

Bakker, A. B., Demerouti, E., & Verbeke, W. (2004). Using the Job Demands–Resources model to predict burnout and performance. *Human Resource Management*, *43*(1), 83–104.

Bakker, A. B., Killmer, C. H., Siegrist, J., & Schaufeli, W. B. (2000). Effort–reward imbalance and burnout among nurses. *Journal of Advanced Nursing*, *31*(4), 884–891.

Bakker, A. B., Schaufeli, W. B., Leiter, M. P., & Taris, T. W. (2008). Work engagement: An emerging concept in occupational health psychology. *Work & Stress*, *22*(3), 187–200.

Berg, J. M., Dutton, J. E., & Wrzesniewski, A. (2013). Job crafting and meaningful work. B. J. Buonocore, F., Agrifoglio, R., & de Gennaro, D. (2021). The role of digital competencies and creativity for job crafting in public administration. In C. Metallo, M. Ferrara, A. Lazazzara, & S. Za (Eds.), *Digital transformation and human behavior: Innovation for people and organisations* (pp. 87–97). Springer. ISBN: 978-30-30475-38-3. https://doi.org/10.1007/978-3-030-47539-0_7

Bourbonnais, R., Comeau, M., Vezina, M., & Dion, G. (1999). Job strain, psychological distress, and burnout in nurses. *American Journal of Industrial Medicine*, *35*(6), 595–606.

Briganti, P., de Gennaro, D., Buonocore, F., & Varriale, L. (2023). Job (dis-) satisfaction in pay-for-performance health care contexts: A meta-synthesis of qualitative literature. *International Journal of Public Sector Management*, *36*(6/7), 606–631. https://doi.org/10.1108/IJPSM-02-2023-0061

Buonocore, F., de Gennaro, D., Lazazzara, A., & Salvatore, D. (2021). How public managers craft their job? A proposal for a JC intervention in the public sector. Impresa Progetto. *Electronic Journal of Management*, *3*, 1–20. ISSN: 1824-3576. https://doi.org/10.15167/1824-3576/IPEJM2021.3.1403

Buonocore, F., de Gennaro, D., Russo, M., & Salvatore, D. (2020). Cognitive job crafting: A possible response to increasing job insecurity and declining professional prestige. *Human Resource Management Journal*, *30* (2), 244–259. ISSN: 1748-8583. https://doi.org/10.1111/1748-8583.12270

Buonocore, F., Russo, M., & de Gennaro, D. (2022). Coping with organizational changes due to executives' succession: The role of personal and contextual resources for job crafting. *International Journal of Public Sector Management*, *36*(1), 64–78. ISSN: 0951-3558. https://doi.org/10.1108/IJPSM-03-2022-0085

Carver, C. S., Scheier, M. F., & Weintraub, J. K. (1989). Assessing coping strategies: A theoretically based approach. *Journal of Personality and Social Psychology*, *56*(2), 267–283.

Csikszentmihalyi, M. (1990). *Flow: The psychology of optimal experience*. Harper & Row.

Cummings, G. G., Tate, K., Lee, S., Wong, C. A., Paananen, T., Micaroni, S. P., & Chatterjee, G. E. (2018). Leadership styles and outcome patterns for the nursing workforce and work environment: A systematic review. *International Journal of Nursing Studies*, *85*, 19–60.

Dall'Ora, C., Griffiths, P., Ball, J., Simon, M., & Aiken, L. H. (2015). Association of 12 h shifts and nurses' job satisfaction, burnout and intention to leave: Findings from a cross-sectional study of 12 European countries. *BMJ Open*, *5*(9), e008331.

de Gennaro, D. (2019). *Job crafting: The art of redesigning a job*. Emerald Publishing Ltd. ISBN: 978-18-38672-22-5, eISBN: 978-18-38672-19-5. https://doi.org/10.1108/9781838672195

de Gennaro, D., Loia, F., & Piscopo, G. (2022). Working role of women in a pandemic world: A poetic inquiry. *Management Research Review*, *45*(11), 1373–1392. ISSN: 2040-8269. https://doi.org/10.1108/MRR-06-2021-0430

de Gennaro, D., & Marino, M. (2024). *Global classroom: Multicultural approaches and organizational strategies in teaching and learning business and economics*. Emerald Publishing Limited. ISBN: 978-1-83549-285-7, eISBN: 978-1-83549-284-0. https://doi.org/10.1108/9781835492840

de Jonge, J., Dollard, M. F., Dormann, C., Le Blanc, P. M., & Houtman, I. L. D. (2000). The Demand–Control model: Specific demands, specific control, and well-defined groups. *International Journal of Stress Management*, *7*(4), 269–287.

Demerouti, E. (2014). Design your own job through job crafting. *European Psychologist*, *19*(4), 237–247.

Demerouti, E., Bakker, A. B., Nachreiner, F., & Schaufeli, W. B. (2001). The Job Demands–Resources model of burnout. *Journal of Applied Psychology*, *86*(3), 499–512.

Edmondson, A. C. (2019). *The fearless organization: Creating psychological safety in the workplace for learning, innovation, and growth*. Wiley.

Epstein, E. G., & Hamric, A. B. (2009). Moral distress, moral residue, and the crescendo effect. *Journal of Clinical Ethics*, *20*(4), 330–342.

Fletcher, D., & Sarkar, M. (2013). Psychological resilience: A review and critique of definitions, concepts, and theory. *European Psychologist*, *18*(1), 12–23.

Folkman, S., Lazarus, R. S., Dunkel-Schetter, C., DeLongis, A., & Gruen, R. J. (1986). Dynamics of a stressful encounter: Cognitive appraisal, coping, and encounter outcomes. *Journal of Personality and Social Psychology*, *50*(5), 992–1003.

Folkman, S., & Moskowitz, J. T. (2004). Coping: Pitfalls and promise. *Annual Review of Psychology*, *55*(1), 745–774.

Grace, P. J., & VanHeuvelen, J. S. (2019). Occupational identity and moral distress in critical care nurses. *Nursing Ethics*, *26*(4), 1191–1205.

Hart, P. L., Brannan, J. D., & De Chesnay, M. (2014). Resilience in nurses: An integrative review. *Journal of Nursing Management*, *22*(6), 720–734.

Healy, C. M., & McKay, M. F. (2000). Nursing stress: The effects of coping strategies and job satisfaction in a sample of Australian nurses. *Journal of Advanced Nursing*, *31*(3), 681–688.

Huang, L., Lei, W., Xu, F., Liu, H., & Yu, L. (2020). Emotional responses and coping strategies in nurses and nursing students during COVID-19 outbreak: A comparative study. *PLoS One*, *15*(8), e0237303.

Karasek, R. A. (1979). Job demands, job decision latitude, and mental strain: Implications for job redesign. *Administrative Science Quarterly*, *24* (2), 285–308.

Karasek, R., & Theorell, T. (1990). *Healthy work: Stress, productivity, and the reconstruction of working life*. Basic Books.

Kristof-Brown, A. L., Zimmerman, R. D., & Johnson, E. C. (2005). Consequences of individuals' fit at work: A meta-analysis of person–job, person–organization, person–group, and person–supervisor fit. *Personnel Psychology*, *58*(2), 281–342.

Laschinger, H. K. S., & Finegan, J. (2005). Empowering nurses for work engagement and health in hospital settings. *The Journal of Nursing Administration*, *35*(10), 439–449.

Lazarus, R. S. (1999). *Stress and emotion: A new synthesis*. Springer.

Lazarus, R. S., & Folkman, S. (1984). *Stress, appraisal, and coping*. Springer.

Lazazzara, A., Tims, M., & de Gennaro, D. (2020). The process of reinventing a job: A meta-synthesis of qualitative job crafting research. *Journal of Vocational Behavior*, *116*(b), 1–18. ISSN: 0001-8791. https://doi.org/10.1016/j.jvb.2019.01.001

Leana, C., Appelbaum, E., & Shevchuk, I. (2009). Work process and quality of care in early childhood education: The role of job crafting. *Academy of Management Journal, 52*(6), 1169–1192.

LeBlanc, V. R. (2009). The effects of acute stress on performance: Implications for health professions education. *Academic Medicine, 84*(10), S25–S33.

Lengnick-Hall, C. A., Beck, T. E., & Lengnick-Hall, M. L. (2011). Developing a capacity for organizational resilience through strategic human resource management. *Human Resource Management Review, 21*(3), 243–255.

Li, J., Yang, W., Cho, S. I., & Haratani, T. (2014). Effort–reward imbalance at work and job dissatisfaction in Chinese healthcare workers: Findings from a cross-sectional study. *International Archives of Occupational and Environmental Health, 87*(3), 239–247.

Linzer, M., Visser, M. R., Oort, F. J., Smets, E. M., McMurray, J. E., & de Haes, H. C. (2000). Predicting and preventing physician burnout: results from the United States and the Netherlands. *The American Journal of Medicine, 111*(2), 170–175.

Mark, G., & Smith, A. P. (2012). Occupational stress, job characteristics, coping, and the mental health of nurses. *British Journal of Health Psychology, 17*(3), 505–521.

Maunder, R. G., Heeney, N. D., Kiss, A., Hunter, J. J., Jeffs, L., Ginty, L., Wiesenfeld, L., Vytelingum, B., Tannenbaum, D. W., & Mazzulli, T. (2021). Psychological impact of the COVID-19 pandemic on hospital workers over time: relationships to occupational role, living with children and elders, and modifiable factors. *General Hospital Psychiatry, 71*, 88–94.

McGrath, A., Reid, N., & Boore, J. (2003). Occupational stress in nursing. *International Journal of Nursing Studies, 40*(5), 555–565.

Mealer, M., Jones, J., Newman, J., McFann, K. K., Rothbaum, B., & Moss, M. (2012). The presence of resilience is associated with a healthier psychological profile in intensive care unit nurses: Results of a national survey. *International Journal of Nursing Studies, 49*(3), 292–299.

Mesmer-Magnus, J., Glew, D. J., & Viswesvaran, C. (2012). A meta-analysis of positive humor in the workplace. *Journal of Managerial Psychology, 27*(2), 155–190.

Peter, R., Alfredsson, L., Hammar, N., Siegrist, J., Theorell, T., & Westerholm, P. (1998). High effort, low reward, and cardiovascular risk factors in employed Swedish men and women: Baseline results from the WOLF study. *Journal of Epidemiology & Community Health*, *52*(9), 540–547.

Petrou, P., Demerouti, E., Peeters, M. C. W., Schaufeli, W. B., & Hetland, J. (2012). Crafting a job on a daily basis: Contextual correlates and the link to work engagement. *Journal of Organizational Behavior*, *33*(8), 1120–1141.

Petrou, P., Demerouti, E., & Schaufeli, W. B. (2015). Job crafting in changing organizations: Antecedents and implications for exhaustion and performance. *Journal of Occupational Health Psychology*, *20*(4), 470–480.

Poncet, M. C., Toullic, P., Papazian, L., Kentish-Barnes, N., Timsit, J. F., Pochard, F., Chevret, S., Schlemmer, B., & Azoulay, E. (2007). Burnout syndrome in critical care nursing staff. *American Journal of Respiratory and Critical Care Medicine*, *175*(7), 698–704.

Riemma, F., Buonocore, F., & de Gennaro, D. (2025). Coping with pressure: Stress management and organizational support in healthcare settings. *Personnel Review*. ahead-of-print. https://doi.org/10.1108/PR-04-2025-0387

Rudolph, C. W., Katz, I. M., Lavigne, K. N., & Zacher, H. (2017). Job crafting: A meta-analysis of relationships with individual differences, job characteristics, and work outcomes. *Journal of Vocational Behavior*, *102*, 112–138.

Rushton, C. H. (2018). *Moral resilience: Transforming moral suffering in healthcare*. Oxford University Press.

Salanova, M., Bakker, A. B., & Llorens, S. (2006). Flow at work: Evidence for an upward spiral of personal and organizational resources. *Journal of Happiness Studies*, *7*(1), 1–22.

Schwarzer, R., & Hallum, S. (2008). Perceived teacher self-efficacy as a predictor of job stress and burnout: Mediation analyses. *Applied Psychology*, *57*, 152–171.

Serrano-Ripoll, M. J., Meneses-Echavez, J. F., Ricci-Cabello, I., Fraile-Navarro, D., Fiol-deRoque, M. A., Pastor-Moreno, G., Castro, A., Ruiz-Pérez, I., Campos, R. Z., & Gonçalves-Bradley, D. C. (2020). Impact of viral epidemic outbreaks on mental health of healthcare workers: A rapid systematic review and meta-analysis. *Journal of Affective Disorders, 277*, 347–357.

Shanafelt, T. D., Sloan, J. A., & Habermann, T. M. (2009). The well-being of physicians. *American Journal of Medicine, 114*(6), 513–519.

Shanafelt, T. D., & Noseworthy, J. H. (2017). Executive leadership and physician well-being: Nine organizational strategies to promote engagement and reduce burnout. *Mayo Clinic Proceedings, 92*(1), 129–146.

Shaukat, N., Ali, D. M., & Razzak, J. (2020). Physical and mental health impacts of COVID-19 on healthcare workers: A scoping review. *International Journal of Emergency Medicine, 13*(1), 40.

Siegrist, J. (1996). Adverse health effects of high-effort/low-reward conditions. *Journal of Occupational Health Psychology, 1*(1), 27–41.

Slišković, A. (2017). Life satisfaction and burnout among healthcare professionals: The mediating role of perceived stress. *Journal of Clinical Psychology in Medical Settings, 24*(3–4), 263–271.

Theorell, T., & Karasek, R. (1996). Current issues relating to psychosocial job strain and cardiovascular disease research. *Journal of Occupational Health Psychology, 1*(1), 9–26.

Tims, M., Bakker, A. B., & Derks, D. (2012). Development and validation of the job crafting scale. *Journal of Vocational Behavior, 80*(1), 173–186.

Tims, M., Bakker, A. B., & Derks, D. (2013). The impact of job crafting on job demands, job resources, and well-being. *Journal of Occupational Health Psychology, 18*(2), 230–240.

Tomo, A., & de Gennaro, D. (2020). Accountants' behavioural reactions to external threats: The mediating role of proactive personality in the goal orientation process. *Meditari Accountancy Research, 29*(6), 1337–1353. ISSN: 2049-372X. https://doi.org/10.1108/MEDAR-04-2020-0843

Tyler, P., & Cushway, D. (1995). Stress in nurses: The effects of coping and social support. *Stress Medicine, 11*(3), 243–251.

Van Bogaert, P., Clarke, S., Willems, R., & Mondelaers, M. (2013). Staff engagement as a target for managing work environments in psychiatric hospitals: Implications for workforce stability and quality of care. *Journal of Clinical Nursing, 22*(11–12), 1717–1728.

Van der Doef, M., & Maes, S. (1999). The Job Demand–Control model and psychological well-being: A review of 20 years of empirical research. *Work & Stress*, *13*(2), 87–114.

van Vegchel, N., de Jonge, J., Bosma, H., & Schaufeli, W. (2005). Reviewing the effort–reward imbalance model: Drawing up the balance of 45 empirical studies. *Social Science & Medicine*, *60*(5), 1117–1131.

van Wingerden, J., Bakker, A. B., & Derks, D. (2017). Fostering employee well-being via a job crafting intervention. *Journal of Vocational Behavior*, *100*, 164–174.

van Wingerden, J., & Poell, R. F. (2019). Meaningful work and resilience among teachers: The mediating role of work engagement and job crafting. *PLoS One*, *14*(9), e0222518.

Vogt, K., Hakanen, J. J., Brauchli, R., Jenny, G. J., & Bauer, G. F. (2016). The consequences of job crafting: A three-wave study. *European Journal of Work & Organizational Psychology*, *25*(3), 353–362.

West, M., Bailey, S., & Williams, E. (2020). *The courage of compassion: Supporting nurses and midwives to deliver high-quality care*. The King's Fund.

Wrzesniewski, A., & Dutton, J. E. (2001). Crafting a job: Revisioning employees as active crafters of their work. *Academy of Management Review*, *26*(2), 179–201.

Xanthopoulou, D., Bakker, A. B., Demerouti, E., & Schaufeli, W. B. (2007). The role of personal resources in the Job Demands–Resources model. *International Journal of Stress Management*, *14*(2), 121–141.

Zhang, Y., Wang, C., Pan, W., Zheng, J., Gao, J., Huang, X., & Cai, S. (2021). Stress, burnout, and coping strategies of frontline nurses during the COVID-19 epidemic in Wuhan and Shanghai, China. *Frontiers in Psychiatry*, *11*, 565520.

Part II

INSIDE THE EXPERIENCE OF HEALTHCARE PROFESSIONALS

INTRODUCTION

The first part of this book outlined the structural and theoretical foundations of stress in healthcare, showing why this sector is uniquely exposed to pressure and why traditional models, though useful, require critical adaptation. Yet to fully grasp the nature of stress in healthcare, we must go beyond models and statistics and turn to the voices of those who live this reality on a daily basis. *Part II brings us inside the experience of healthcare professionals*, exploring their perceptions, narratives and coping strategies through the lens of empirical research.

This section is based on an in-depth qualitative study conducted with *41 healthcare professionals*, including physicians, nurses and allied health staff. Semi-structured interviews allowed participants to reflect openly on their daily routines, the sources of stress they encounter and the strategies they employ to cope with such pressures. The design of the study prioritised depth over breadth: by listening carefully to individual experiences, the research team sought to capture the complexity, ambivalence and nuance that often escape large-scale surveys.

The interviews were systematically transcribed and analysed using *thematic analysis*, a method particularly suited to uncovering recurrent patterns while also preserving the richness of subjective accounts. Four thematic clusters emerged:

- *Sources of stress*, ranging from excessive workload and staff shortages to emotional demands, organisational inefficiencies and ethical dilemmas.

- *Coping strategies*, which varied from problem-focused adjustments to emotion-focused practices, as well as more proactive behaviours like job crafting and peer support.
- *Enabling and hindering factors*, highlighting how organisational culture, leadership and team dynamics can either amplify stress or provide crucial buffers.
- *Outcomes for professionals and organisations*, showing how individual well-being and patient care are inextricably linked.

By bringing these themes to light, Part II situates theoretical discussions within the *lived world of healthcare work*. The professionals' accounts not only validate but also challenge existing stress models. They illustrate, for instance, how stress is rarely the product of a single factor but emerges from the interplay of structural shortages, interpersonal tensions and moral conflicts. They also reveal how coping is not a solitary endeavour but often a collective and relational process, shaped by team dynamics and organisational support.

Crucially, these narratives remind us that behind every policy debate and theoretical model are *human beings striving to care for others while also struggling to care for themselves*. By entering their experience, we gain insight into both the fragility and resilience of healthcare systems. We also see more clearly how organisational practices, leadership choices and cultural contexts can determine whether stress becomes destructive or whether it can be managed, reframed and even transformed into opportunities for growth.

The chapters that follow will present the findings of this study in detail, illustrating them with direct quotations from participants and situating them within the broader literature. They will also serve as a foundation for rethinking stress models in Part III and for deriving actionable strategies in Part IV. In this way, Part II is the *empirical heart of the book*: it takes us inside the lived experience of stress and coping in healthcare, and in doing so, it grounds the rest of the discussion in the realities of those most directly affected.

3

LISTENING TO THE FRONTLINE: STORIES OF PRESSURE AND COPING

ABSTRACT

This chapter gives voice to healthcare professionals by exploring the lived experience of stress and coping through qualitative evidence from frontline practice. Drawing on semi-structured interviews with 41 healthcare professionals across roles and settings, and supported by illustrative case vignettes, this chapter adopts an interpretive approach that privileges depth and meaning-making. The methodological design allows stress to be examined not merely as an objective condition but as a subjective and relational experience shaped by organisational, ethical and emotional dynamics.

The findings identify three interrelated clusters of stressors: chronic workload intensity and staff shortages, the emotional labour inherent in patient care and ethical dilemmas associated with resource scarcity and moral distress. These stressors rarely operate in isolation; rather, they accumulate and interact, producing compounding effects that heighten vulnerability to burnout and disengagement. This chapter then examines coping strategies across three levels. At the individual level, professionals draw on personal resources such as resilience, self-regulation and problem-solving. At the collective level, team dynamics, peer support, humour and informal debriefing emerge as critical buffers against stress. However, the analysis also reveals significant organisational blind spots, where responsibility for coping is implicitly shifted onto individuals and teams while structural drivers of stress remain unaddressed.

By highlighting the tensions between personal agency, collective coping and organisational accountability, this chapter underscores the limits of individual-centred approaches to stress management. It concludes that sustainable coping in healthcare requires integrated interventions that align individual, team and organisational levels, recognising stress as a systemic rather than purely personal phenomenon.

Keywords: Frontline healthcare experiences; qualitative research; emotional labour; moral distress; collective coping

3.1 METHODOLOGICAL APPROACH: INTERVIEWS AND CASE VIGNETTES

Understanding the lived experiences of healthcare professionals requires methodological choices that privilege depth, nuance and context. Quantitative surveys and standardised instruments, while useful for establishing prevalence and correlations, often fail to capture the complexity of how stress is experienced, interpreted and managed by individuals working in dynamic organisational settings. For this reason, the research presented in this book (see Riemma et al., 2025) employed a *qualitative approach*, rooted in semi-structured interviews and enriched by the development of *case vignettes*.

3.1.1 Semi-Structured Interviews

The central methodological tool was a series of *semi-structured interviews* with 41 healthcare professionals across different roles and settings. Participants included physicians, nurses and other allied health staff, ensuring that diverse perspectives were represented. The sample was designed to reflect variation in professional seniority, clinical specialisation and organisational context. This diversity allowed for the identification of both recurring patterns and role-specific nuances in the experience of stress.

The interview guide was informed by the literature on stress and coping (Bakker & Demerouti, 2007; Lazarus & Folkman, 1984), as well as by practical concerns identified in the healthcare management field. Core questions asked participants to reflect on:

- the *daily pressures* and stressors they faced in their professional lives;
- the *strategies* they employed to cope with such stress, including both individual and collective practices;

- the *role of organisational support*, leadership and culture in shaping their experiences;
- the *perceived consequences* of stress and coping for both professional well-being and the quality of patient care.

Interviews were conducted in a flexible manner, allowing participants to elaborate on themes they found most salient. This flexibility ensured that the voices of participants drove the research agenda rather than being constrained by overly rigid categories.

3.1.2 Data Collection and Analysis

The interviews were conducted both face-to-face and online, depending on feasibility and participant availability. All sessions were recorded with informed consent, transcribed verbatim and anonymised to protect confidentiality. The corpus of transcripts was then analysed using *thematic analysis*, following Braun and Clarke's (2006) widely recognised six-phase framework: familiarisation with the data, generating initial codes, searching for themes, reviewing themes, defining and naming themes and producing the report.

Through this process, the research team identified four overarching thematic domains:

- *Sources of stress*, such as workload intensity, staff shortages and moral distress.
- *Coping strategies*, ranging from problem-focused tactics (e.g., task reorganisation, peer collaboration) to emotion-focused practices (e.g., meditation, distancing).
- *Enabling and hindering factors*, highlighting the decisive role of leadership, organisational culture and available resources.
- *Consequences*, illustrating the reciprocal relationship between stress, coping, staff well-being and patient outcomes.

This inductive approach allowed the findings to emerge directly from the data, while still being informed by the theoretical frameworks discussed in Part I.

3.1.3 Case Vignettes

In addition to thematic patterns, the study developed *case vignettes* to bring individual stories to life. These vignettes are condensed narratives, drawn from interviews, that illustrate the complexities and contradictions of stress in healthcare. They serve several purposes:

- *Illustrative*: showing how abstract themes (e.g., 'lack of recognition') manifest in the lived reality of a nurse or physician.
- *Analytical*: highlighting the interplay of multiple stressors and coping strategies within a single professional trajectory.
- *Communicative*: making the research accessible and relatable, particularly for policymakers and managers who may not be familiar with qualitative analysis.

Each vignette is based on one or more interviews but carefully anonymised and sometimes combined to protect confidentiality. For example, one vignette may portray a mid-career nurse balancing excessive patient loads with creative job crafting strategies (de Gennaro, 2019), while another may describe a physician struggling with moral distress during the pandemic but finding relief in collegial solidarity. By embedding these narratives, the book aims to *humanise data*, grounding abstract analysis in tangible, recognisable experiences.

3.1.4 Methodological Rationale

The choice of semi-structured interviews and vignettes reflects a deliberate epistemological stance: that understanding stress in healthcare requires not only measuring its frequency but also *listening to stories*. As scholars such as Kvale (1996) and Riessman (2008) argue, interviews are not neutral data-gathering tools but co-constructed narratives that reveal how individuals make sense of their experiences. In this research, participants were not treated merely as respondents but as *knowledge holders*, whose insights enrich both theory and practice.

Moreover, the qualitative approach complements the theoretical frameworks discussed in earlier chapters. The Transactional Model of Stress and Coping emphasises appraisal processes; interviews provide direct access to how professionals articulate these appraisals. The Job Demands–Resources model highlights the balance between demands and resources; case vignettes illustrate how this balance is negotiated in practice. Thus, methodology and theory are not separate but mutually reinforcing.

3.1.5 Limitations and Strengths

No methodological choice is without limitations. Qualitative interviews, by their nature, cannot claim statistical generalisability. The findings are context-bound, reflecting the particular organisational and cultural environments of the participants. However, the goal was not generalisation but *transferability*: providing insights that resonate across settings while acknowledging their situated nature (Lincoln & Guba, 1985). The strength of this approach lies in its ability to capture nuance, contradiction and emotional depth – dimensions often invisible in quantitative studies.

3.2 KEY STRESSORS IDENTIFIED: WORKLOAD, EMOTIONAL LABOUR, ETHICAL DILEMMAS

The qualitative study conducted with 41 healthcare professionals offered a rich and multi-layered picture of the pressures experienced in everyday practice (see also Riemma et al., 2025). Thematic analysis revealed three clusters of stressors that were most consistently reported across roles and settings: *workload intensity and staff shortages*, *emotional labour and relational demands* and *ethical dilemmas linked to resource scarcity and moral distress*. While these categories are analytically distinct, they often overlap in practice, producing cumulative effects that heighten the risk of burnout and erode professional well-being.

The most salient stressor reported by participants was the chronic intensity of workload. Physicians and nurses described excessive patient loads, unpredictable demands and administrative burdens that left little time for recovery. As one participant noted: *'There are days when I feel like I am running a marathon without ever crossing the finish line. Patients keep coming, documentation keeps piling up, and there is no space to breathe.'* Such testimonies echo findings from international research showing that high workload and insufficient staffing ratios are strongly associated with burnout, medical errors and turnover (Aiken et al., 2002; Dall'Ora et al., 2020).

Importantly, workload stress was not perceived merely as a question of volume but also of *time pressure and fragmentation*. Professionals described the stress of 'task-switching,' being forced to juggle multiple responsibilities without the chance to focus deeply on patient care. Documentation and bureaucratic requirements emerged as a specific source of frustration, reinforcing earlier evidence that electronic health records and reporting systems, while designed to improve efficiency, often increase administrative load and reduce time available for patient interaction (Shanafelt et al., 2016).

The second major stressor was the *emotional labour* inherent in healthcare work. Following Hochschild's (1983) classic definition, emotional labour refers to the regulation of feelings and expressions to fulfil the emotional requirements of a job. Healthcare professionals are expected to display empathy, patience and compassion, even in the face of suffering, anger or hostility. Participants highlighted the toll of constantly managing their own emotions while simultaneously absorbing the distress of patients and families.

> *One nurse described: 'When a patient cries, you cannot cry with them. You must remain calm, reassure them, and then carry all those feelings inside yourself.' Another participant emphasized the cumulative effect of repeated exposure to death and suffering: 'You try to stay strong, but after years of watching patients die, it eats away at you. It doesn't leave when you go home.'*

Research confirms that emotional labour is a predictor of emotional exhaustion and compassion fatigue (Brotheridge & Grandey, 2002; Zapf, 2002). Yet it is also a source of meaning and professional pride, underscoring the ambivalence of this stressor. The very same empathic connection that fuels motivation can, under conditions of inadequate support, become overwhelming. Studies of 'compassion fatigue' in nursing, for instance, highlight how persistent emotional demands without adequate recovery time lead to disengagement, cynicism and burnout (Figley, 2002; Peters, 2018).

A third cluster of stressors emerged around *ethical dilemmas*, particularly in situations where professionals felt constrained from providing the care they believed was appropriate. This aligns with the concept of *moral distress*, first introduced by Jameton (1984), describing the psychological disequilibrium that arises when individuals know the right course of action but are unable to act due to institutional barriers.

Several participants spoke of the anguish of having to ration care or prioritise among patients due to staff shortages and limited resources: *'It is devastating when you know what the patient needs but the resources are not there. You feel you are betraying your professional oath.'* Others described conflicts between professional judgement and organisational protocols, which sometimes forced them to compromise on what they saw as best for the patient.

Moral distress has been widely documented as a source of burnout, turnover and reduced quality of care (Epstein & Hamric, 2009; Rushton, 2018). It is particularly acute in high-intensity settings such as intensive care units, oncology or palliative care, where life-and-death decisions intersect with systemic constraints. The narratives from this study confirm that ethical dilemmas are not abstract philosophical puzzles but lived stressors with profound psychological and organisational consequences.

While workload, emotional labour and ethical dilemmas can be analytically distinguished, participants' accounts made clear that these stressors often interact in compounding ways. Excessive workload reduces the time available to provide empathic care, which in turn intensifies emotional strain and moral conflict. Ethical dilemmas are experienced more acutely when professionals are already depleted by heavy workloads and emotional demands. As one physician summarised: *'It's not one thing – it's everything together. The pressure of time, the emotions you carry, and the knowledge that sometimes you cannot do what is right. That combination is what breaks you.'*

This interdependence highlights the systemic nature of stress in healthcare. It is not reducible to isolated variables but emerges from a nexus of organisational structures, interpersonal dynamics and ethical tensions. Addressing stress therefore requires integrated strategies that simultaneously tackle workload management, provide support for emotional labour and create environments where ethical concerns can be voiced and addressed.

3.3 COPING STRATEGIES: PERSONAL RESOURCES, TEAM DYNAMICS, AND ORGANISATIONAL BLIND SPOTS

The interviews conducted with 41 healthcare professionals revealed not only the intensity of stressors but also the multiple ways in which individuals and groups attempt to cope with them. Coping emerged as a multidimensional phenomenon, spanning personal strategies rooted in psychological resources, collective processes embedded in teams and professional communities and – tellingly – organisational contexts that often failed to provide adequate support. This section explores these three dimensions in depth: *personal resources*, *team dynamics* and *organisational blind spots*.

3.3.1 Personal Resources: The Role of Agency and Resilience

Many professionals described strategies aimed at maintaining equilibrium at an individual level (see also Riemma et al., 2025). These ranged from classical *problem-focused coping*, such as reorganising tasks, prioritising under pressure and creating personal checklists, to *emotion-focused coping*, such as practicing mindfulness, physical exercise or compartmentalising distress after shifts. One physician reflected: *'I try to remind myself that I can only do what is humanly possible. At the end of the day, I make a list of what I achieved, instead of obsessing over what I couldn't.'*

The literature confirms that *personal resources* – such as self-efficacy, optimism and resilience – play a critical role in buffering the effects of stress. Hobfoll's (1989) Conservation of Resources theory suggests that individuals draw on and protect key resources to withstand stress. In healthcare, personal strategies like mindfulness-based stress reduction (Krasner et al., 2009) and resilience training (McAllister & McKinnon, 2009) have been shown to reduce burnout and improve emotional regulation. However, the interviews also revealed limits: self-care strategies, while useful, often felt insufficient when systemic pressures were overwhelming. As one nurse put it, *'You can meditate or run as much as you want, but if every day you face twice as many patients as you can handle, it only helps so much.'*

3.3.2 Team Dynamics: Collective Coping and Peer Support

Beyond individual strategies, coping often emerged as a *collective endeavour* rooted in teamwork, collegiality and informal peer support. Many participants emphasised that colleagues provided the most immediate and reliable buffer against stress. One nurse stated: *'When I feel like I'm drowning, it's usually a colleague who pulls me up – sometimes just with a joke, sometimes by taking over a task.'* Humour, informal debriefing and solidarity during difficult shifts were repeatedly cited as essential.

This resonates with research on *social support* as a protective factor in high-demand occupations (Viswesvaran et al., 1999). Team-based coping mechanisms – such as shared decision-making, collective sensemaking after critical incidents and peer mentoring – enhance not only well-being but also clinical outcomes (West et al., 2018). Concepts such as *collective resilience* (Lengnick-Hall et al., 2011) and *psychological safety* (Edmondson, 1999) are particularly relevant: when team members feel safe to express vulnerabilities and rely on each other, stress is more effectively managed and errors are reduced.

Yet the interviews also revealed fragility in these dynamics. Supportive teams were not universally present; in some contexts, competition, hierarchical distance or interpersonal conflicts eroded collective coping. As one junior physician lamented: *'If you make a mistake, some colleagues will help you learn, others will make you feel small. That difference changes everything.'* Thus, team dynamics can either mitigate stress or exacerbate it, depending on the culture of the unit and the quality of relationships.

3.3.3 Organisational Blind Spots: When Coping Becomes a Private Burden

Perhaps the most striking finding from the interviews was the perception that *organisations often abdicated responsibility for supporting coping*, leaving individuals and teams to manage stress largely on their own. Several participants described a gap between rhetorical commitments to staff well-being and the reality of daily practice. A senior nurse noted: *'They tell us to take care of ourselves, to be resilient, but then they cut staff and increase our shifts. It feels hypocritical.'*

This points to what might be termed *organisational blind spots*: the tendency of healthcare institutions to valorise resilience at the individual level while ignoring structural drivers of stress. Research confirms this pattern. Interventions focused narrowly on individual coping – such as resilience workshops or yoga sessions – often show limited effects when systemic issues like understaffing or excessive administrative load remain unchanged (West et al., 2016). Such 'band-aid' approaches may even backfire by creating the impression that stress is a personal failing rather than an organisational responsibility (Kinman & Grant, 2020).

Organisational blind spots also extend to the recognition of *moral distress*. While individuals and teams develop strategies to endure ethical challenges, without institutional forums for ethical reflection or policy clarity, coping can degenerate into disengagement or cynicism (Epstein & Hamric, 2009). Several professionals reported 'silencing' themselves when faced with untenable decisions, an avoidance strategy that reduces immediate conflict but erodes long-term integrity.

3.3.4 Interactions and Tensions

The interplay of personal, team and organisational levels reveals a paradox. Personal and team strategies can buffer stress in the short term, but without organisational alignment, they risk being *fragile and unsustainable*. Teams that support each other may delay burnout, but chronic understaffing eventually overwhelms even the strongest solidarity. Similarly, personal resilience may sustain professionals temporarily, but without systemic support, resilience turns into resignation.

As one physician poignantly observed: '*We cope because we care, but the system takes advantage of that. They know we won't abandon our patients, so they keep stretching us thinner.*' This insight underscores the need for integrated approaches: coping should be understood not only as individual or collective effort but as a *shared responsibility* involving organisations and policymakers.

REFERENCES

Aiken, L. H., Clarke, S. P., Sloane, D. M., Sochalski, J., & Silber, J. H. (2002). Hospital nurse staffing and patient mortality, nurse burnout, and job dissatisfaction. *JAMA*, *288*(16), 1987–1993.

Bakker, A. B., & Demerouti, E. (2007). The Job Demands–Resources model: State of the art. *Journal of Managerial Psychology*, *22*(3), 309–328.

Braun, V., & Clarke, V. (2006). Using thematic analysis in psychology. *Qualitative Research in Psychology*, *3*(2), 77–101.

Brotheridge, C. M., & Grandey, A. A. (2002). Emotional labor and burnout: Comparing two perspectives of "people work.". *Journal of Vocational Behavior*, *60*(1), 17–39.

Dall'Ora, C., Ball, J., Reinius, M., & Griffiths, P. (2020). Burnout in nursing: A theoretical review. *Human Resources for Health*, *18*(1), 41.

de Gennaro, D. (2019). *Job crafting: The art of redesigning a job*. Emerald Publishing Ltd. ISBN: 978-18-38672-22-5, eISBN: 978-18-38672-19-5. https://doi.org/10.1108/9781838672195

Edmondson, A. (1999). Psychological safety and learning behavior in work teams. *Administrative Science Quarterly*, *44*(2), 350–383.

Epstein, E. G., & Hamric, A. B. (2009). Moral distress, moral residue, and the crescendo effect. *Journal of Clinical Ethics*, *20*(4), 330–342.

Figley, C. R. (2002). *Compassion fatigue: Psychotherapists' chronic lack of self care*. Brunner-Routledge.

Hobfoll, S. E. (1989). Conservation of resources: A new attempt at conceptualizing stress. *American Psychologist*, *44*(3), 513–524.

Hochschild, A. R. (1983). *The managed heart: Commercialization of human feeling*. University of California Press.

Jameton, A. (1984). *Nursing practice: The ethical issues*. Prentice-Hall.

Kinman, G., & Grant, L. (2020). Presenteeism during the COVID-19 pandemic: Risks and solutions. *Occupational Medicine*, *70*(5), 243–244.

Krasner, M. S., Epstein, R. M., Beckman, H., Suchman, A. L., Chapman, B., Mooney, C. J., & Quill, T. E. (2009). Association of an educational program in mindful communication with burnout, empathy, and attitudes among primary care physicians. *JAMA*, *302*(12), 1284–1293.

Kvale, S. (1996). *InterViews: An introduction to qualitative research interviewing*. Sage.

Lazarus, R. S., & Folkman, S. (1984). *Stress, appraisal, and coping*. Springer.

Lengnick-Hall, C. A., Beck, T. E., & Lengnick-Hall, M. L. (2011). Developing a capacity for organizational resilience through strategic human resource management. *Human Resource Management Review*, *21*(3), 243–255.

Lincoln, Y. S., & Guba, E. G. (1985). *Naturalistic inquiry*. Sage.

McAllister, M., & McKinnon, J. (2009). The importance of teaching and learning resilience in the health disciplines: A critical review of the literature. *Nurse Education Today*, *29*(4), 371–379.

Peters, E. (2018). Compassion fatigue in nursing: A concept analysis. *Nursing Forum*, *53*(4), 466–480.

Riemma, F., Buonocore, F., & de Gennaro, D. (2025). Coping with pressure: Stress management and organizational support in healthcare settings. *Personnel Review. ahead-of-print*. https://doi.org/10.1108/PR-04-2025-0387

Riessman, C. K. (2008). *Narrative methods for the human sciences*. Sage.

Rushton, C. H. (2018). *Moral resilience: Transforming moral suffering in healthcare*. Oxford University Press.

Shanafelt, T. D., Dyrbye, L. N., & West, C. P. (2016). Addressing physician burnout: The way forward. *JAMA, 317*(9), 901–902.

Viswesvaran, C., Sanchez, J. I., & Fisher, J. (1999). The role of social support in the process of work stress: A meta-analysis. *Journal of Vocational Behavior, 54*(2), 314–334.

West, C. P., Dyrbye, L. N., Erwin, P. J., & Shanafelt, T. D. (2016). Interventions to prevent and reduce physician burnout: A systematic review and meta-analysis. *The Lancet, 388*(10057), 2272–2281.

West, M., Eckert, R., Collins, B., & Chowla, R. (2018). *Caring to change: How compassionate leadership can stimulate innovation in health care*. The King's Fund.

Zapf, D. (2002). Emotion work and psychological well-being: A review of the literature and some conceptual considerations. *Human Resource Management Review, 12*(2), 237–268.

4

WHAT ORGANISATIONS GET WRONG (AND RIGHT) ABOUT STRESS

ABSTRACT

This chapter examines how healthcare organisations shape stress and coping, highlighting both common organisational failures and promising practices. Drawing on qualitative evidence from frontline professionals, it argues that stress in healthcare is not merely an individual phenomenon but a structural and cultural outcome strongly influenced by leadership, organisational culture and material conditions of work. This chapter contrasts command-and-control leadership styles with compassionate leadership, showing how hierarchical, compliance-driven approaches tend to exacerbate stress by silencing staff voices and undermining psychological safety, whereas compassionate leadership fosters trust, recognition and collective resilience.

The analysis then explores organisational culture as a double-edged force. Cultures characterised by openness, solidarity and learning can buffer extreme pressures and sustain resilience, while cultures of silence, stigma and blame normalise suffering and inhibit both coping and organisational learning. Importantly, this chapter highlights the paradox whereby cultures of resilience may compensate for systemic failures, inadvertently shifting the burden of adaptation onto frontline professionals.

Finally, this chapter reveals the often-hidden role of organisational structures, staffing levels and technology in shaping everyday stress. Chronic understaffing, bureaucratic workflows and poorly implemented digital technologies emerge as powerful stress amplifiers, constraining professional autonomy and intensifying moral distress. Using the Job Demands–Resources framework as an interpretive lens, this chapter demonstrates that sustainable stress management requires more than individual resilience or cultural change alone. It concludes that meaningful organisational responses to stress must integrate compassionate leadership, supportive cultures and structural reforms that rebalance demands and resources, aligning staff well-being with the long-term sustainability of healthcare systems.

Keywords: Compassionate leadership; organisational culture; psychological safety; staffing and workload; healthcare organisational stress

4.1 THE ROLE OF LEADERSHIP: FROM COMMAND-AND-CONTROL TO COMPASSIONATE LEADERSHIP

Among the most powerful themes to emerge from the narratives of healthcare professionals was the decisive role that leadership plays in shaping experiences of stress and well-being. Time and again, participants emphasised that leadership was not a neutral background factor but a central determinant of whether pressures became overwhelming or manageable, whether coping strategies were sustained or eroded and whether teams experienced resilience or collapse. Leadership sets the tone of organisational culture, influences the quality of interpersonal relationships and communicates the extent to which staff well-being is recognised as a legitimate priority alongside patient outcomes.

The interviews revealed a widespread tension between two paradigms of leadership. On one side, many professionals described enduring the legacies of *command-and-control leadership*, characterised by rigid hierarchies, limited voice and a focus on compliance and efficiency. This model, while historically dominant in healthcare systems, was experienced as amplifying stress rather than alleviating it. Participants recounted situations where managers imposed unrealistic targets without consultation, discouraged open discussion of errors and responded to staff distress with admonitions to 'be professional' or 'toughen up.' As one nurse reflected, '*When leadership means just giving orders and pushing us to meet numbers, it feels like we are machines, not people. That kind of leadership makes stress unbearable.*'

This command-and-control style resonates with the literature documenting the limitations of authoritarian leadership in complex professional contexts. Research shows that directive, punitive styles of leadership are associated with higher burnout, lower job satisfaction and increased turnover intentions in healthcare (Cummings et al., 2018; Wong et al., 2013). The high-pressure environment of hospitals may create temptations for managers to centralise control and tighten oversight (see Loia et al., 2022), but such strategies often backfire by undermining autonomy and eroding trust (Riemma et al., 2025). Instead of reducing uncertainty, they add an additional layer of stress by silencing staff voices and diminishing psychological safety.

Against this backdrop, participants also described a contrasting model: *compassionate leadership*. Compassionate leaders were not those who ignored performance demands but those who combined accountability with empathy, authority with listening and vision with humility. A recurring phrase in the interviews was 'being seen.' As one physician stated, '*What makes the difference is when leaders really see you – not just as someone filling a shift, but as a person with limits, with emotions, with a life outside the hospital.*' Professionals emphasised the profound impact of seemingly small acts: leaders who checked in personally after a traumatic incident, who recognised effort publicly or who simply acknowledged fatigue and made space for recovery.

This resonates strongly with a growing body of scholarship on *compassionate and inclusive leadership* in healthcare. West et al. (2017, 2020) argue that compassionate leadership – defined as attending, understanding, empathising and helping – is not a soft add-on but a critical enabler of innovation, safety and resilience. Leaders who create environments of psychological safety allow staff to raise concerns, admit mistakes and seek support without fear of retribution (Edmondson, 2019). The evidence is clear: in settings where staff feel heard and valued, burnout rates decline, engagement rises and patient outcomes improve (Shanafelt & Noseworthy, 2017).

The COVID-19 pandemic offered particularly stark illustrations of the contrast between these models (de Gennaro et al., 2022). Several participants recalled leaders who remained distant during the crisis, communicating only directives via email, or emphasising targets without acknowledging the extraordinary strain staff were under. Others, however, spoke of leaders who demonstrated visibility and solidarity – being physically present onwards, taking time to listen and openly acknowledging uncertainty. One nurse recalled: '*What helped us through those months was not policies on paper, but a director who came every day, asked how we were holding up, and stayed until the last patient was discharged. That gave us strength.*'

The transition from command-and-control to compassionate leadership is not merely about style; it is about reimagining the very purpose of leadership in healthcare. Command-and-control assumes that leaders' primary role is to enforce compliance and maximise efficiency. Compassionate leadership, by contrast, assumes that leaders' role is to enable the conditions under which staff can perform effectively and sustainably. This includes ensuring adequate resources, fostering cultures of respect and inclusion and modelling behaviours that normalise vulnerability and care. Far from undermining performance, such leadership enhances it by aligning staff well-being with organisational goals.

Yet the interviews also revealed barriers to this transition. Some professionals expressed scepticism that compassionate leadership could survive in systems dominated by cost pressures, bureaucratic requirements and performance metrics. Others noted inconsistencies between leaders' words and actions: '*They talk about well-being in meetings, but then they cut shifts and increase the workload. That contradiction makes people cynical.*' These tensions highlight the danger of reducing compassion to rhetoric or symbolic gestures. Compassionate leadership requires structural alignment: policies that back up rhetoric with resources, evaluation systems that reward supportive behaviours and organisational cultures that sustain, rather than punish, leaders who prioritise humanity alongside efficiency.

The movement towards compassionate leadership is also connected to broader shifts in organisational theory and practice. Healthcare, as a high-pressure, knowledge-intensive sector, exemplifies the limits of mechanistic models of management. Complexity theory suggests that adaptive, participatory forms of leadership are better suited to dynamic systems where uncertainty and interdependence are the norm (Uhl-Bien & Arena, 2018). Compassionate leadership aligns with this by creating space for dialogue, learning and adaptation. Moreover, in professions where meaning and identity are central motivators, leadership that affirms purpose and dignity is more effective than leadership that reduces professionals to interchangeable units.

In sum, the findings from this study reinforce the growing recognition that leadership is a *critical lever* in addressing stress and burnout in healthcare. Command-and-control leadership exacerbates pressure by silencing voices and prioritising compliance over humanity. Compassionate leadership, by contrast, transforms stress from an isolating burden into a shared challenge, enabling resilience at both individual and collective levels. The transition between these paradigms is neither automatic nor easy; it requires deliberate commitment, structural support and cultural change (de Gennaro & Marino, 2023). But as the voices of healthcare professionals make clear, the stakes are high. Leadership, perhaps more than any other factor, determines whether healthcare systems remain locked in cycles of burnout and attrition or move towards sustainability, resilience and humane care.

4.2 ORGANISATIONAL CULTURE AND ITS DOUBLE EDGE: RESILIENCE VS. SILENCE

If leadership provides the visible face of organisational life, culture constitutes its less tangible but equally decisive foundation. Organisational culture shapes how stress is perceived, how coping is legitimised and how professionals relate to both their work and one another. In the interviews conducted with healthcare professionals, organisational culture repeatedly emerged as a *double-edged phenomenon.* On the one hand, cultures characterised by solidarity, openness and learning were powerful enablers of resilience, allowing staff to endure extraordinary pressures without collapsing (Riemma et al., 2025). On the other hand, cultures marked by hierarchy, stigma and silence not only failed to buffer stress but also actively exacerbated it, creating climates where suffering was normalised and voices were muted.

Participants often described the ambivalence of culture with striking clarity. One nurse remarked: *'In our unit, when something bad happens, we debrief together. We talk, we cry, we laugh. That is what keeps us going.'* In another setting, however, a physician offered a very different account: *'Here, if you admit you are struggling, they look at you as if you are weak. Everyone knows people are burning out, but nobody says it out loud.'* These narratives underscore the *dual potential of culture*: it can sustain resilience or enforce silence, empower or marginalise, humanise or dehumanise.

The literature provides ample support for this duality. Positive organisational cultures – those that encourage psychological safety, mutual support and continuous learning – are associated with lower burnout, higher engagement and improved patient safety (Edmondson, 1999; Nembhard & Edmondson, 2006). Conversely, toxic cultures characterised by blame, stigma or rigid hierarchy create conditions where stress festers, moral distress intensifies and attrition accelerates (Kahn, 1990; West et al., 2018). Healthcare, with its strong traditions of professional hierarchy and implicit expectations of stoicism, is particularly vulnerable to the silencing effects of culture.

The *resilience dimension* of culture was vividly illustrated in accounts of teams where compassion and solidarity were not only permitted but also celebrated. Professionals described rituals of informal debriefing, shared humour and collective adaptation in crises. One participant recalled the early months of the COVID-19 pandemic: *'We had nothing – no masks, no clear protocols. What saved us was the way we held each other up. Even in the worst days, we felt like a family.'* Such cultures embody what Sutcliffe and Vogus (2003) call 'organizational resilience,' the collective capacity to absorb strain and adapt under pressure. They reinforce not only coping but also meaning, enabling professionals to reframe adversity as a shared challenge rather than an isolated struggle.

Yet resilient cultures can sometimes mask deeper vulnerabilities. As scholars caution, resilience can become *an ideology* that valorises endurance while obscuring systemic deficiencies (Joseph, 2013). Several participants noted that solidarity within teams often compensated for chronic under-staffing and managerial neglect. '*We support each other, yes – but sometimes it feels like we are patching holes that leadership refuses to fix,*' said one nurse. In this sense, cultures of resilience risk being co-opted by organisations as a substitute for structural investment, effectively shifting the burden of adaptation onto frontline staff.

The *silence dimension* of culture was equally prominent. Silence operated in two main forms: *defensive silence*, where staff withheld concerns out of fear of negative consequences and *acquiescent silence*, where staff disengaged due to a sense of futility (Morrison & Milliken, 2000). Several professionals described environments where raising concerns about workload or patient safety was discouraged, implicitly or explicitly. One junior doctor commented: '*You learn quickly not to complain. If you do, you are told that everyone else is managing, so why can't you?*' Such silencing not only undermines individual well-being but also erodes organisational learning, as valuable information about risks and failures never surfaces.

The coexistence of resilience and silence within the same organisational cultures highlights their *paradoxical nature*. Some teams managed to create micro-cultures of openness and solidarity even within broader institutions that discouraged dissent. Conversely, cultures that appeared cohesive on the surface sometimes masked widespread suffering that was never articulated. This paradox illustrates the need to look beyond surface-level indicators of 'team spirit' to critically examine whether cultures genuinely support well-being or merely normalise silent endurance.

From a theoretical perspective, these findings resonate with the distinction between *engaged coping cultures* and *defensive coping cultures* (Kahn & Heaphy, 2014). In engaged coping cultures, stress is acknowledged collectively, emotions are legitimised and coping is shared. In defensive coping cultures, stress is privatised, emotional expression is stigmatised and silence becomes the dominant norm. The organisational consequences are profound: the former fosters resilience and innovation, while the latter fuels burnout, turnover and compromised care quality.

The voices of professionals make clear that organisational culture cannot be treated as a soft or peripheral issue. Culture is a *structural determinant* of how stress is experienced and managed. Efforts to build sustainable healthcare systems must therefore confront culture directly: rewarding openness rather than silence, embedding compassion rather than stoicism and ensuring that resilience is not a substitute for systemic investment but a complement to it. As one participant concluded poignantly: '*We don't need a culture that teaches us how to survive stress – we need one that makes survival less necessary.*'

4.3 THE HIDDEN ROLE OF STRUCTURES, STAFFING AND TECHNOLOGY IN SHAPING STRESS

While discussions of stress in healthcare often focus on individual resilience or interpersonal dynamics, the narratives of professionals collected in this study make it clear that *organisational structures, staffing configurations and technological systems* exert a profound, though sometimes hidden, influence on daily experiences of pressure (Riemma et al., 2025). Stress does not emerge in a vacuum: it is shaped by the ways in which work is organised, resources are allocated and tools are designed and implemented. Structures may either enable sustainable practice or create environments where even the most resilient individuals and teams are stretched beyond their limits.

One of the most consistent themes in the interviews concerned *staffing shortages* and their cascading effects. Professionals repeatedly described the experience of working in understaffed wards, where ratios of patients to nurses or physicians made it impossible to provide adequate care. As one nurse explained: '*Even before the pandemic, we were always short. You end up running, cutting corners, feeling guilty. The stress is not just from the pace but from knowing you are not giving patients what they deserve.*' These experiences resonate with robust evidence showing that inadequate staffing is directly associated with higher burnout, lower job satisfaction and worse patient outcomes (Aiken et al., 2002; Briganti et al., 2023; Dall'Ora et al., 2020). Staffing shortages force professionals into a state of *chronic overload*, where the impossibility of meeting demands creates not only physical fatigue but also moral distress.

Organisational *structures and workflows* were also described as amplifiers of stress. Several participants highlighted the rigidity of bureaucratic protocols and the inefficiencies of fragmented systems. A physician noted: '*We spend hours filling out forms and double-checking things in three different platforms. It feels like the system is designed to waste our time.*' Such frustrations reflect what Shanafelt et al. (2016) call the 'clerical burden' of healthcare: the excessive documentation requirements that divert attention from patient care and erode professional satisfaction. In contexts where workflows are poorly coordinated, professionals are caught in a constant cycle of interruptions, duplications and delays, which exacerbate stress and reduce the sense of control over one's work.

Technology emerged in the interviews as a particularly *ambivalent factor*. On the one hand, digital tools such as electronic health records, telemedicine platforms and automated monitoring systems were recognised as potentially supportive resources. Some participants described the relief of having quick access to patient histories or the flexibility of remote consultations. On the other hand, technology often intensified stress when poorly designed or implemented without adequate training. One participant observed: *'The computer takes longer to understand than the patient. You spend ten minutes clicking and the patient is waiting. It's stressful because it feels like the system comes first, not the person.'*

This ambivalence mirrors findings from the literature on healthcare digitalisation. While digital tools can enhance coordination and safety, they often add to workloads and reduce autonomy when usability is low (Buntin et al., 2011; Wachter, 2015). The 'technological paradox' in healthcare thus becomes evident: tools intended to streamline care may, if not carefully adapted, create new layers of complexity and stress. Moreover, technology can reconfigure professional identities, as algorithmic decision-making and predictive analytics sometimes challenge clinicians' sense of autonomy and expertise (Greenhalgh et al., 2019). For some, this provoked feelings of alienation: *'I studied for years to make decisions, but now I feel like I'm just validating what the computer tells me.'*

The hidden role of structures, staffing and technology also underscores the *systemic nature of stress*. Stress is not only a psychological reaction but also a structural outcome, produced by the interaction of organisational arrangements and resource allocation. For example, insufficient staffing intersects with rigid workflows to create chronic time pressure, which is then compounded by technological inefficiencies. Professionals may attempt to cope individually or collectively, but the underlying causes remain embedded in structures. As one interviewee summarised: *'They tell us to take care of ourselves, but it's the system that is sick. Until that changes, our stress will not go away.'*

From a theoretical perspective, these findings resonate with the Job Demands–Resources (JD-R) model (Bakker & Demerouti, 2007). Staffing shortages and bureaucratic inefficiencies represent excessive *demands*, while supportive structures and well-designed technologies could act as *resources*.

Yet in practice, the balance is often skewed, with demands vastly outweighing resources. The hidden role of organisational structures becomes evident precisely because these factors are often invisible in everyday discourse on coping: stress is framed as an individual matter, while systemic contributors remain unaddressed.

Importantly, structural and technological issues also shape the *possibility of resilience*. In organisations with adequate staffing, streamlined workflows and supportive technologies, personal and team coping strategies can flourish. In contrast, when structures are dysfunctional, resilience becomes fragile, as professionals expend energy compensating for systemic deficiencies rather than building sustainable practices. This reinforces the argument that resilience should not be romanticised as an individual trait but recognised as dependent on *structural conditions* that organisations must actively create.

In conclusion, the accounts of healthcare professionals make clear that leadership and culture, though critical, cannot be disentangled from the *material realities of structures, staffing and technology*. These elements, often overlooked in stress discourse, constitute the hidden architecture that shapes daily work. If healthcare systems are to move towards sustainability, they must confront these systemic determinants directly: ensuring adequate staffing ratios, redesigning workflows to minimise bureaucratic inefficiencies and implementing technology that serves both patients and professionals. Without such structural reforms, even the most committed leaders and supportive cultures will struggle to transform stress from a corrosive force into an opportunity for resilience and renewal.

REFERENCES

Aiken, L. H., Clarke, S. P., Sloane, D. M., Sochalski, J., & Silber, J. H. (2002). Hospital nurse staffing and patient mortality, nurse burnout, and job dissatisfaction. *JAMA, 288*(16), 1987–1993.

Bakker, A. B., & Demerouti, E. (2007). The job demands–resources model: State of the art. *Journal of Managerial Psychology, 22*(3), 309–328.

Briganti, P., de Gennaro, D., Buonocore, F., & Varriale, L. (2023). Job (dis-) satisfaction in pay-for-performance health care contexts: A meta-synthesis of qualitative literature. *International Journal of Public Sector Management, 36*(6/7), 606–631. https://doi.org/10.1108/IJPSM-02-2023-0061

Buntin, M. B., Burke, M. F., Hoaglin, M. C., & Blumenthal, D. (2011). The benefits of health information technology: A review of the recent literature shows predominantly positive results. *Health Affairs*, *30*(3), 464–471.

Cummings, G. G., Tate, K., Lee, S., Wong, C. A., Paananen, T., Micaroni, S. P., & Chatterjee, G. E. (2018). Leadership styles and outcome patterns for the nursing workforce and work environment: A systematic review. *International Journal of Nursing Studies*, *85*, 19–60.

Dall'Ora, C., Ball, J., Reinius, M., & Griffiths, P. (2020). Burnout in nursing: A theoretical review. *Human Resources for Health*, *18*(1), 41.

de Gennaro, D., Loia, F., & Piscopo, G. (2022). Working role of women in a pandemic world: A poetic inquiry. *Management Research Review*, *45*(11), 1373–1392. ISSN: 2040-8269. https://doi.org/10.1108/MRR-06-2021-0430

de Gennaro, D., & Marino, M. (2023). *Cross-cultural undergraduate internships: A toolkit for empowering the next generation*. Emerald Publishing Limited. ISBN: 978-1-80455-357-2, eISBN: 978-1-80455-356-5. https://doi.org/10.1108/9781804553565

Edmondson, A. (1999). Psychological safety and learning behavior in work teams. *Administrative Science Quarterly*, *44*(2), 350–383.

Edmondson, A. C. (2019). *The fearless organization: Creating psychological safety in the workplace for learning, innovation, and growth*. Wiley.

Greenhalgh, T., Wherton, J., Papoutsi, C., Lynch, J., & Hughes, G. (2019). Infrastructure revisited: An ethnographic case study of how health information infrastructure shapes and constrains technological innovation. *Journal of Medical Internet Research*, *21*(12), e16093.

Joseph, J. (2013). Resilience as embedded neoliberalism: A governmentality approach. *Resilience*, *1*(1), 38–52.

Kahn, W. A. (1990). Psychological conditions of personal engagement and disengagement at work. *Academy of Management Journal*, *33*(4), 692–724.

Kahn, W. A., & Heaphy, E. D. (2014). *Relational contexts of personal engagement at work*. In A. B. Bakker (Ed.), *Advances in positive organizational psychology* (pp. 163–179). Emerald Publishing Limited.

Loia, F., de Gennaro, D., & Adinolfi, P. (2022). Managerial hubristic-behavioral strategy: How to cope with chaotic and uncertain contexts. *Management Research Review*, *45*(9), 1137–1154. ISSN: 2040-8269. https://doi.org/10.1108/MRR-11-2021-0811

Morrison, E. W., & Milliken, F. J. (2000). Organizational silence: A barrier to change and development in a pluralistic world. *Academy of Management Review*, *25*(4), 706–725.

Nembhard, I. M., & Edmondson, A. C. (2006). Making it safe: The effects of leader inclusiveness and professional status on psychological safety and improvement efforts in health care teams. *Journal of Organizational Behavior*, *27*(7), 941–966.

Riemma, F., Buonocore, F., & de Gennaro, D. (2025). Coping with pressure: Stress management and organizational support in healthcare settings. *Personnel Review. ahead-of-print.* https://doi.org/10.1108/PR-04-2025-0387

Shanafelt, T. D., Dyrbye, L. N., & West, C. P. (2016). Addressing physician burnout: The way forward. *JAMA*, *317*(9), 901–902.

Shanafelt, T. D., & Noseworthy, J. H. (2017). Executive leadership and physician well-being: Nine organizational strategies to promote engagement and reduce burnout. *Mayo Clinic Proceedings*, *92*(1), 129–146.

Sutcliffe, K. M., & Vogus, T. J. (2003). *Organizing for resilience*. In K. S. Cameron, J. E. Dutton, & R. E. Quinn (Eds.), *Positive organizational scholarship* (pp. 94–110). Berrett-Koehler.

Uhl-Bien, M., & Arena, M. (2018). Leadership for organizational adaptability: A theoretical synthesis and integrative framework. *The Leadership Quarterly*, *29*(1), 89–104.

Wachter, R. M. (2015). *The digital doctor: Hope, hype, and harm at the dawn of medicine's computer age*. McGraw-Hill.

West, C. P., Dyrbye, L. N., Erwin, P. J., & Shanafelt, T. D. (2017). Interventions to prevent and reduce physician burnout: A systematic review and meta-analysis. *The Lancet*, *388*(10057), 2272–2281.

West, M., Bailey, S., & Williams, E. (2020). *The courage of compassion: Supporting nurses and midwives to deliver high-quality care*. The King's Fund.

West, M., Eckert, R., Collins, B., & Chowla, R. (2018). *Caring to change: How compassionate leadership can stimulate innovation in health care*. The King's Fund.

Wong, C. A., Cummings, G. G., & Ducharme, L. (2013). The relationship between nursing leadership and patient outcomes: A systematic review update. *Journal of Nursing Management*, *21*(5), 709–724.

Part III

RETHINKING MODELS AND PRACTICES

INTRODUCTION

The preceding chapters have traced the contours of stress in healthcare, from its defining pressures to the theoretical models that have shaped our understanding for decades. What emerges is a complex but consistent picture: healthcare is not only a high-pressure environment but one where traditional models of stress, while useful, are often insufficient to capture the lived realities of professionals and the systemic challenges of organisations. Stress in healthcare is neither a transient episode nor a purely individual phenomenon. It is deeply embedded in organisational structures, cultural expectations and the reciprocal relationships between workers, patients and institutions.

Part III – Rethinking Models and Practices turns this recognition into a deliberate agenda for change. It asks: how can existing theories be expanded to account for the unique demands of healthcare? What role should organisations play in complementing individual coping strategies with systemic support? And, perhaps most critically, how can healthcare systems move beyond short-term fixes to cultivate long-term resilience and sustainability?

In this part, we go beyond the established frameworks of the Transactional Model, the Demand–Control paradigm and the Effort–Reward Imbalance model. While these models have generated valuable insights, they often focus on the individual professional as the locus of stress and coping. In practice, however, healthcare stress is rarely experienced in isolation. It unfolds within teams, institutions and wider systems shaped by policy, leadership and resource allocation. Rethinking stress in healthcare therefore requires a dual shift: from *individual to collective* and from *reactive coping to proactive organisational design*.

The chapters that follow explore this rethinking in two ways. Chapter 5 examines how healthcare findings can expand existing theories, highlighting where traditional models fall short and how they might be enriched by concepts such as collective resilience, moral distress and systemic adaptation. Chapter 6 then translates these insights into concrete organisational practices, identifying actionable strategies for managers and leaders to foster healthier workplaces and more sustainable care systems.

Taken together, this part of the book argues that the future of stress management in healthcare depends on *integration*: the integration of theory and practice, of individual resilience and organisational responsibility, and of short-term interventions with long-term systemic reform. Only by embracing this integrated perspective can healthcare organisations hope to address the profound and enduring pressures faced by their workforce while safeguarding the quality of patient care.

5

EXPANDING STRESS AND COPING FRAMEWORKS

ABSTRACT

This chapter advances stress and coping theory by integrating organisational and sector-specific insights derived from healthcare settings. It argues that classic models of occupational stress remain foundational but insufficient when applied to highly complex, team-based and ethically charged environments such as healthcare. This chapter demonstrates how incorporating organisational support strengthens these models, particularly by reshaping appraisal processes, buffering high demands and restoring social reciprocity under conditions of chronic strain.

A central contribution of this chapter is the reconceptualisation of resilience. Moving beyond individualistic framings, the analysis redefines resilience as a collective, relational and systemic capacity emerging from team dynamics, organisational culture, leadership and value alignment. Evidence from healthcare practice shows that individual coping skills are necessary but inadequate in the absence of supportive structures, psychological safety and institutional recognition. This chapter critiques managerial approaches that overemphasise individual resilience training while neglecting structural drivers of stress, such as understaffing, moral distress and bureaucratic overload.

Finally, this chapter outlines how healthcare enriches general stress theories through sector-specific adaptations. Emotional labour, moral distress, interprofessional teamwork, system-level constraints and vocational meaning are identified as core dimensions that require explicit theoretical integration. By incorporating these elements, stress and coping frameworks become more multidimensional and better suited to guiding both research and organisational interventions. This chapter concludes that healthcare is not merely an application context but a source of theoretical innovation, pushing stress models towards more ethical, collective and system-oriented perspectives.

Keywords: Organisational support; collective resilience; Job Demands–Resources model; moral distress; healthcare-specific stress theory

5.1 INTEGRATING ORGANISATIONAL SUPPORT INTO CLASSIC STRESS MODELS

Classic stress models such as the *Transactional Model of Stress and Coping* (Lazarus & Folkman, 1984), the *Demand–Control model* (Karasek, 1979; Karasek & Theorell, 1990) and the *Effort–Reward Imbalance model* (Siegrist, 1996) have provided invaluable conceptual tools for understanding the antecedents and mechanisms of occupational stress. Yet one limitation that has been repeatedly noted is their relative underemphasis on the *organisational and systemic context* in which stress occurs (Cooper et al., 2001; Semmer, 2007). These models often treat coping and strain primarily as individual phenomena, shaped by personal appraisal, individual resources or perceptions of fairness. However, in healthcare settings – where stress is deeply embedded in team dynamics, organisational culture and systemic resource allocation – the role of *organisational support* emerges as an indispensable dimension.

5.1.1 Organisational Support as a Buffer of Stress

The notion of organisational support has been theorised most directly through *Perceived Organizational Support (POS)*, defined by Eisenberger et al. (1986) as employees' general belief that their organisation values their contributions and cares about their well-being. A vast body of research demonstrates that POS is strongly related to reduced stress and burnout, increased job satisfaction and enhanced organisational commitment (Rhoades & Eisenberger, 2002). In healthcare, where demands are particularly high and resources often scarce, POS functions as a critical buffer against the deleterious effects of stress (Caesens et al., 2016; Haar & Roche, 2010).

Integrating POS into the *Transactional Model* highlights how organisational support can reshape both *primary appraisal* (by framing stressors as challenges rather than threats) and *secondary appraisal* (by expanding perceived coping resources). For example, a physician facing overwhelming caseloads may perceive the situation as less threatening if their hospital leadership demonstrates flexibility, provides additional staff or openly acknowledges the strain. Similarly, access to mentoring, peer support or wellness resources expands the range of coping options available, making stress more manageable (Shanafelt & Noseworthy, 2017).

5.1.2 Extending the Demand–Control Model

The *Demand–Control model* suggests that strain is most likely when workers face high demands with low decision latitude (Karasek, 1979). However, healthcare professionals often operate in environments where control is structurally limited – protocols, safety regulations and hierarchical decision-making constrain autonomy even when expertise is high. In such contexts, *organisational support* becomes a crucial third dimension, supplementing the Demand–Control–Support extension (Johnson & Hall, 1988).

Research confirms that organisational support significantly moderates the relationship between job demands and strain in healthcare. Bourbonnais et al. (1999) found that nurses with low autonomy but high supervisory support reported significantly lower psychological distress than those without support. Similarly, Van der Doef and Maes (1999), in their review of 20 years of Demand–Control research, concluded that the buffering role of support is particularly salient in high-strain jobs such as healthcare. This suggests that while individual autonomy may be constrained, supportive management practices and collegial relationships can mitigate the adverse effects of high demands.

5.1.3 Extending the Effort–Reward Imbalance (ERI) Model

The *ERI model* (Siegrist, 1996) conceptualises stress as arising when the high efforts expended by workers are not matched by commensurate rewards, including financial compensation, recognition and career opportunities. Here too, organisational support plays a pivotal role. Recognition from leaders, respect from colleagues and opportunities for professional development are not merely ‘nice to have’ extras but core components of the social reciprocity underpinning healthy work.

Healthcare research provides strong empirical support for this perspective. Li et al. (2014) found that Chinese nurses experiencing high ERI but also reporting high organisational support were less likely to develop depressive symptoms. Van Vegchel et al. (2005), in their comprehensive review of ERI studies, similarly concluded that supportive leadership and recognition attenuate the negative impact of effort-reward imbalance on health outcomes. Integrating organisational support into ERI thus strengthens the model's explanatory power by acknowledging the institutional mechanisms that can restore balance even under demanding conditions.

5.1.4 Towards a Multi-level Understanding

Integrating organisational support into classic stress models also aligns with the *Job Demands–Resources (JD-R) framework* (Bakker & Demerouti, 2007; Demerouti et al., 2001), which explicitly positions resources – structural, social and personal – as central to understanding stress and motivation. Organisational support can be understood as a critical *job resource*, one that directly buffers the health-impairment process and fuels the motivational process. Studies show that in healthcare, organisational support not only reduces burnout but also fosters work engagement, resilience and patient-centred care (Cummings et al., 2018; West et al., 2020).

Furthermore, organisational support contributes to *collective resilience* by shaping team climate and psychological safety (Edmondson, 2019). In environments where errors are stigmatised and staff feel unsupported, stress escalates and learning opportunities are lost. By contrast, organisations that cultivate supportive cultures encourage open communication, shared problem-solving and mutual trust, all of which mitigate stress at the collective level.

5.2 NEW INSIGHTS FROM HEALTHCARE: REDEFINING RESILIENCE AS COLLECTIVE, NOT JUST INDIVIDUAL

Resilience has traditionally been conceptualised as an *individual trait or capacity*, referring to the ability to adapt positively to adversity, maintain functioning under pressure and recover quickly from setbacks (Fletcher & Sarkar, 2013). This framing, however, risks overemphasising personal characteristics such as optimism, self-efficacy or emotional regulation, while underplaying the social and organisational contexts in which stress unfolds.

Healthcare, perhaps more than any other sector, demonstrates the limitations of this individual-centred view (Riemma et al., 2025). The extreme demands of clinical practice – life-or-death decision-making, continuous exposure to suffering, moral dilemmas and resource scarcity – cannot be met through individual resilience alone. Instead, the healthcare environment points to the importance of *collective resilience*, a capacity embedded in teams, institutions and professional communities.

Recent research suggests that resilience in healthcare should be redefined not as a personal quality but as a *dynamic, relational and systemic phenomenon*. First, resilience emerges through *team-level processes*. Studies show that when healthcare workers perceive strong social support, shared responsibility and open communication within teams, they are better able to withstand stress and avoid burnout (West et al., 2020). Team resilience has been described as 'the capacity of a team to withstand and overcome stressors, to adapt positively, and to maintain effective functioning' (Alliger et al., 2015, p. 177). For example, during the COVID-19 pandemic, multidisciplinary teams in intensive care units reported that coordinated communication, cross-training and mutual trust were essential in sustaining morale and preventing collapse, even under extreme conditions (de Gennaro et al., 2022; Maunder et al., 2021). These findings highlight that resilience is not simply distributed across individuals but is constructed collectively through interaction.

Second, resilience in healthcare is *culturally and organisationally shaped*. Organisational factors such as leadership style, recognition, staffing and safety culture exert powerful influences on whether professionals can adapt effectively to stress. Edmondson's (2019) work on psychological safety demonstrates that teams with supportive leadership and cultures of openness are more resilient because individuals feel safe to voice concerns, report errors and seek help. Conversely, in organisations characterised by blame or silence, individual resilience is insufficient to overcome systemic dysfunction. Resilience, in this view, is not a matter of 'toughening up' workers but of creating environments where adaptive responses are possible and encouraged (Robertson et al., 2015).

Third, collective resilience is sustained through *shared narratives and values*. Healthcare professionals often frame their work in terms of vocation, compassion and service, which provides a moral foundation for enduring hardship (Rushton, 2018). Yet when organisational or policy environments undermine these values – for instance, when cost-cutting compromises patient care – resilience falters and moral distress emerges (Epstein & Hamric, 2009). Collective resilience therefore requires alignment between institutional values and professional identities, ensuring that individuals feel their sacrifices are meaningful and reciprocated. This cultural alignment is as critical as material resources in fostering resilience across the workforce (de Gennaro & Marino, 2023).

The redefinition of resilience as collective also challenges the widespread managerial discourse that emphasises resilience training at the individual level, often through mindfulness, cognitive-behavioural strategies or stress management workshops (Buonocore et al., 2020). While such interventions have documented benefits (Spinelli et al., 2019; West et al., 2016), they risk placing responsibility for resilience solely on the worker, implying that failure to cope reflects personal deficiency rather than systemic imbalance (Kinman & Grant, 2020). In healthcare, where stressors are often structural – such as chronic understaffing, long shifts or bureaucratic overload – such an individualising approach is not only insufficient but potentially counterproductive, as it obscures the organisational accountability for providing adequate support.

Instead, insights from healthcare indicate that resilience must be conceptualised as *multi-level and interdependent*. Individual coping skills are necessary but not sufficient; they must be reinforced by team dynamics, organisational support and professional cultures. This perspective resonates with the JD-R model (Bakker & Demerouti, 2007), which positions resources – social, structural and cultural – as central drivers of resilience and engagement. Healthcare exemplifies this model vividly: when demands are overwhelming but resources are strengthened through supportive leadership, effective teamwork and value alignment, resilience emerges not as a personal trait but as a collective outcome.

In sum, healthcare settings provide compelling evidence that resilience is not best understood as a property of individuals but as a *relational and systemic capacity*. Teams, organisations and professions construct resilience together by sharing responsibility, sustaining values and creating supportive environments. Redefining resilience in these terms represents a crucial step forward for both theory and practice, moving the focus from 'fixing the individual' to transforming the conditions that make resilience sustainable. Only by embracing this collective perspective can healthcare systems hope to build resilience that is not fragile or temporary, but enduring, equitable and integrated into the very fabric of care delivery.

5.3 SECTOR-SPECIFIC ADAPTATIONS: WHAT HEALTHCARE ADDS TO GENERAL THEORIES OF STRESS

The study of occupational stress has benefited greatly from general frameworks such as the Transactional Model of Stress and Coping (Lazarus & Folkman, 1984), the Demand–Control model (Karasek, 1979; Karasek & Theorell, 1990), the ERI model (Siegrist, 1996), and, more recently, the JD-R model (Bakker & Demerouti, 2007; Demerouti et al., 2001). These theories have been validated across multiple industries and professions, offering powerful insights into the mechanisms through which job demands, resources and appraisal processes affect well-being. Yet healthcare provides a *unique context* that challenges and enriches these theories in several important ways. Healthcare work is not only cognitively and emotionally demanding but also ethically charged, team-based and highly scrutinised. As a result, stress in healthcare often manifests in ways that cannot be fully explained by general models without *sector-specific adaptations*.

One distinctive contribution of healthcare is the central role of *emotional labour*. Hochschild's (1983) concept of emotional labour – managing one's emotions to meet organisational expectations – is especially salient in nursing, palliative care and mental health services, where compassion and empathy are core to the role. General stress theories acknowledge emotional demands as job stressors, but healthcare research demonstrates their pervasive and cumulative effects. For instance, Zapf et al. (2001) showed that emotional labour is strongly associated with burnout, particularly emotional exhaustion and depersonalisation, among healthcare staff. This suggests that models of stress in healthcare must explicitly account for the chronic strain of sustained emotional engagement and the risk of compassion fatigue (Figley, 2002; Peters, 2018).

A second unique feature of healthcare stress is the phenomenon of *moral distress*. First defined by Jameton (1984), moral distress occurs when professionals know the ethically appropriate action to take but are unable to act due to institutional or resource constraints. Moral distress has been widely reported among nurses, physicians and allied health workers and has been linked to burnout, turnover and reduced quality of care (Epstein & Hamric, 2009; Rushton, 2018). While general stress models highlight appraisal and control, healthcare research emphasises that stress can be particularly damaging when it undermines professional integrity and identity. This requires theories of stress to incorporate *moral and ethical dimensions*, which are less pronounced in other sectors.

Third, healthcare highlights the importance of *team-based and interprofessional dynamics* in stress processes. Unlike many occupations where stress is primarily individualised, healthcare delivery relies heavily on coordination across professional boundaries. Stressors such as role conflict, poor communication and interprofessional tensions have been shown to significantly predict burnout and job dissatisfaction in healthcare teams (Cummings et al., 2018; Hall, 2005). This suggests that stress models need to move beyond the individual and include *collective stress and coping processes*. Concepts such as team resilience (Alliger et al., 2015) and psychological safety (Edmondson, 2019) become essential to explaining how healthcare teams adapt under pressure (Riemma et al., 2025).

Fourth, healthcare illustrates how *system-level stressors* shape individual experiences. General models often focus on proximal stressors such as workload or control, but healthcare workers operate within highly regulated and resource-constrained systems. Staffing shortages, financial pressures and policy reforms are systemic conditions that continually filter down to the level of individual work. Aiken et al. (2002) demonstrated that higher nurse-to-patient ratios are directly linked not only to burnout among nurses but also to patient mortality, underscoring the systemic nature of stress. Similarly, West et al. (2020) argued that staff well-being is inseparable from healthcare quality, making stress not only an occupational health issue but also a *systemic risk to patient safety and organisational sustainability*.

Finally, healthcare underscores the role of *meaning-making and vocational identity* in stress and resilience. Many healthcare workers enter the profession with strong prosocial motivations and the sense of making a difference often sustains them during adversity (Schaufeli & Bakker, 2004). Yet when organisational conditions undermine these values – through excessive bureaucracy, inadequate recognition or resource rationing – stress takes on existential dimensions, eroding professional purpose and driving attrition (Grace & VanHeuvelen, 2019). This suggests that stress theories applied to healthcare must pay greater attention to *identity, values and meaning*, dimensions less frequently foregrounded in general occupational stress models.

Taken together, these insights indicate that healthcare contributes not just data but also *conceptual refinements* to stress theories. Emotional labour, moral distress, team-based dynamics, systemic constraints and vocational meaning are all distinctive features that enrich our understanding of how stress operates in high-pressure, ethically charged environments. By incorporating these sector-specific dimensions, general stress models become more nuanced and better equipped to guide both research and practice. Healthcare thus serves as both a testing ground and a source of theoretical innovation, pushing stress models to evolve from primarily individual and structural explanations towards more *multidimensional, ethical and systemic accounts.*

REFERENCES

Aiken, L. H., Clarke, S. P., Sloane, D. M., Sochalski, J., & Silber, J. H. (2002). Hospital nurse staffing and patient mortality, nurse burnout, and job dissatisfaction. *JAMA, 288*(16), 1987–1993.

Alliger, G. M., Cerasoli, C. P., Tannenbaum, S. I., & Vessey, W. B. (2015). Team resilience: How teams flourish under pressure. *Organizational Dynamics, 44*(3), 176–184.

Bakker, A. B., & Demerouti, E. (2007). The Job Demands–Resources model: State of the art. *Journal of Managerial Psychology, 22*(3), 309–328.

Bourbonnais, R., Comeau, M., Vezina, M., & Dion, G. (1999). Job strain, psychological distress, and burnout in nurses. *American Journal of Industrial Medicine, 35*(6), 595–606.

Buonocore, F., de Gennaro, D., Russo, M., & Salvatore, D. (2020). Cognitive job crafting: A possible response to increasing job insecurity and declining professional prestige. *Human Resource Management Journal, 30* (2), 244–259. ISSN: 1748-8583. https://doi.org/10.1111/1748-8583.12270

Caesens, G., Stinglhamber, F., & Ohana, M. (2016). Perceived organizational support and well-being: A weekly study. *Journal of Managerial Psychology, 31*(7), 1214–1230.

Cooper, C. L., Dewe, P. J., & O'Driscoll, M. P. (2001). *Organizational stress: A review and critique of theory, research, and applications.* Sage.

Cummings, G. G., Tate, K., Lee, S., Wong, C. A., Paananen, T., Micaroni, S. P., & Chatterjee, G. E. (2018). Leadership styles and outcome patterns for the nursing workforce and work environment: A systematic review. *International Journal of Nursing Studies, 85*, 19–60.

de Gennaro, D., Loia, F., & Piscopo, G. (2022). Working role of women in a pandemic world: A poetic inquiry. *Management Research Review, 45*(11), 1373–1392. ISSN: 2040-8269. https://doi.org/10.1108/MRR-06-2021-0430

de Gennaro, D., & Marino, M. (2023). *Cross-cultural undergraduate internships: A toolkit for empowering the next generation*. Emerald Publishing Limited. ISBN: 978-1-80455-357-2, eISBN: 978-1-80455-356-5. https://doi.org/10.1108/9781804553565

Demerouti, E., Bakker, A. B., Nachreiner, F., & Schaufeli, W. B. (2001). The Job Demands–Resources model of burnout. *Journal of Applied Psychology*, *86*(3), 499–512.

Edmondson, A. C. (2019). *The fearless organization: Creating psychological safety in the workplace for learning, innovation, and growth*. Wiley.

Eisenberger, R., Huntington, R., Hutchison, S., & Sowa, D. (1986). Perceived organizational support. *Journal of Applied Psychology*, *71*(3), 500–507.

Epstein, E. G., & Hamric, A. B. (2009). Moral distress, moral residue, and the crescendo effect. *Journal of Clinical Ethics*, *20*(4), 330–342.

Figley, C. R. (2002). *Compassion fatigue: Psychotherapists' chronic lack of self care*. Brunner-Routledge.

Fletcher, D., & Sarkar, M. (2013). Psychological resilience: A review and critique of definitions, concepts, and theory. *European Psychologist*, *18*(1), 12–23.

Grace, P. J., & VanHeuvelen, J. S. (2019). Occupational identity and moral distress in critical care nurses. *Nursing Ethics*, *26*(4), 1191–1205.

Haar, J. M., & Roche, M. (2010). Family supportive organization perceptions and employee outcomes: The mediating effects of life satisfaction. *International Journal of Human Resource Management*, *21*(7), 999–1014.

Hall, P. (2005). Interprofessional teamwork: Professional cultures as barriers. *Journal of Interprofessional Care*, *19*(S1), 188–196.

Hochschild, A. R. (1983). *The managed heart: Commercialization of human feeling*. University of California Press.

Jameton, A. (1984). *Nursing practice: The ethical issues*. Prentice-Hall.

Johnson, J. V., & Hall, E. M. (1988). Job strain, work place social support, and cardiovascular disease: A cross-sectional study of a random sample of the Swedish working population. *American Journal of Public Health*, *78* (10), 1336–1342.

Karasek, R. A. (1979). Job demands, job decision latitude, and mental strain: Implications for job redesign. *Administrative Science Quarterly, 24* (2), 285–308.

Karasek, R., & Theorell, T. (1990). *Healthy work: Stress, productivity, and the reconstruction of working life.* Basic Books.

Kinman, G., & Grant, L. (2020). Presenteeism during the COVID-19 pandemic: Risks and solutions. *Occupational Medicine*, *70*(5), 243–244.

Lazarus, R. S., & Folkman, S. (1984). *Stress, appraisal, and coping.* Springer.

Li, J., Yang, W., Cho, S. I., & Haratani, T. (2014). Effort–reward imbalance at work and depressive symptoms in Chinese healthcare workers. *International Archives of Occupational and Environmental Health*, *87*(3), 239–247.

Maunder, R. G., Heeney, N. D., Kiss, A., Hunter, J. J., Jeffs, L., Ginty, L. Wiesenfeld, L., Vytelingum, B., Tannenbaum, D. W., & Mazzulli, T. (2021). Psychological impact of the COVID-19 pandemic on hospital workers over time: Relationships to occupational role, living with children and elders, and modifiable factors. *General Hospital Psychiatry*, *71*, 88–94.

Peters, E. (2018). Compassion fatigue in nursing: A concept analysis. *Nursing Forum*, *53*(4), 466–480.

Rhoades, L., & Eisenberger, R. (2002). Perceived organizational support: A review of the literature. *Journal of Applied Psychology*, *87*(4), 698–714.

Riemma, F., Buonocore, F., & de Gennaro, D. (2025). Coping with pressure: Stress management and organizational support in healthcare settings. *Personnel Review. ahead-of-print.* https://doi.org/10.1108/PR-04-2025-0387

Robertson, I. T., Cooper, C. L., Sarkar, M., & Curran, T. (2015). Resilience training in the workplace from 2003 to 2014: A systematic review. *Journal of Occupational and Organizational Psychology*, *88*(3), 533–562.

Rushton, C. H. (2018). *Moral resilience: Transforming moral suffering in healthcare.* Oxford University Press.

Schaufeli, W. B., & Bakker, A. B. (2004). Job demands, job resources, and their relationship with burnout and engagement: A multi-sample study. *Journal of Organizational Behavior*, *25*(3), 293–315.

Semmer, N. K. (2007). Recognition and respect as basic needs: The case of occupational stress. *Psychotherapy and Psychosomatics*, *76*(3), 123–128.

Shanafelt, T. D., & Noseworthy, J. H. (2017). Executive leadership and physician well-being: Nine organizational strategies to promote engagement and reduce burnout. *Mayo Clinic Proceedings*, *92*(1), 129–146.

Siegrist, J. (1996). Adverse health effects of high-effort/low-reward conditions. *Journal of Occupational Health Psychology*, *1*(1), 27–41.

Spinelli, C., Wisener, M., & Khoury, B. (2019). Mindfulness training for healthcare professionals and trainees: A meta-analysis of randomized controlled trials. *Journal of Psychosomatic Research*, *120*, 29–38.

Van der Doef, M., & Maes, S. (1999). The job Demand–Control(-Support) model and psychological well-being: A review of 20 years of empirical research. *Work & Stress*, *13*(2), 87–114.

Van Vegchel, N., de Jonge, J., Bosma, H., & Schaufeli, W. B. (2005). Reviewing the effort–reward imbalance model: Drawing up the balance of 45 empirical studies. *Social Science & Medicine*, *60*(5), 1117–1131.

West, M., Bailey, S., & Williams, E. (2020). *The courage of compassion: Supporting nurses and midwives to deliver high-quality care*. The King's Fund.

West, C. P., Dyrbye, L. N., Erwin, P. J., & Shanafelt, T. D. (2016). Interventions to prevent and reduce physician burnout: A systematic review and meta-analysis. *The Lancet*, *388*(10057), 2272–2281.

Zapf, D., Seifert, C., Schmutte, B., Mertini, H., & Holz, M. (2001). Emotion work and job stressors and their effects on burnout. *Psychology and Health*, *16*(5), 527–545.

6

DESIGNING HEALTHIER ORGANISATIONS

ABSTRACT

This chapter translates theoretical insights on stress and coping into actionable strategies for designing healthier healthcare organisations. It argues that sustainable stress reduction requires a shift from reactive, individual-centred interventions towards systemic, evidence-based organisational design. This chapter first examines workforce planning and workload management as foundational levers for well-being, highlighting robust evidence linking staffing levels, skill mix and workload distribution to burnout, patient safety and organisational sustainability. Workforce planning is framed as a strategic responsibility rather than a purely technical function.

This chapter then reviews leadership practices shown to mitigate stress, emphasising transformational, authentic, compassionate and shared leadership models. These approaches are presented as mechanisms for fostering psychological safety, fairness and engagement, particularly in high-pressure and uncertain environments. Attention is also given to practical interventions, including staff support programmes, peer networks and digital tools, illustrating how formalised support and technology can enhance collective resilience when thoughtfully implemented. Beyond discrete interventions, this chapter underscores the importance of organisational learning and continuous feedback loops. Well-being is conceptualised as a dynamic system property that requires ongoing monitoring, reflection and adaptation, rather than episodic initiatives. Finally, this chapter highlights the often-overlooked role of physical spaces, recovery rituals, empowerment and co-design. By involving healthcare professionals in shaping workflows, environments and decision-making processes, organisations can embed recovery, dignity and voice into everyday practice.

Keywords: Workforce planning; leadership for well-being; organisational learning; staff support interventions; co-design; empowerment

6.1 WORKFORCE PLANNING AND WORKLOAD MANAGEMENT

Effective workforce planning and workload management lie at the very heart of stress mitigation in healthcare organisations. While much of the occupational stress literature emphasises individual coping and organisational culture, there is strong empirical evidence that structural issues – particularly staffing levels, skill mix and workload distribution – are among the most significant predictors of burnout, job dissatisfaction and turnover (Aiken et al., 2002; Shanafelt et al., 2012). Workforce planning is therefore not merely a technical exercise in human resources management but a strategic intervention with direct implications for employee well-being, patient safety and organisational sustainability.

6.1.1 The Scale of the Workforce Challenge

Healthcare systems worldwide face chronic workforce shortages, exacerbated by demographic shifts, increased demand for services and the ageing of the health workforce itself (World Health Organization, 2016, 2020). The WHO projects a shortfall of more than 10 million health workers globally by 2030, particularly in low- and middle-income countries, but shortages are also severe in high-income contexts (Campbell et al., 2013). These gaps directly translate into increased workload, longer shifts and greater stress for existing staff. Research consistently demonstrates that inadequate staffing is one of the strongest predictors of burnout among both nurses and physicians (Aiken et al., 2012; Dall'Ora et al., 2015).

Beyond absolute shortages, *maldistribution* of staff further contributes to stress. Rural areas and underserved communities often lack adequate numbers of healthcare professionals, forcing providers to work beyond safe capacity. Skill mix imbalances – such as over-reliance on junior staff or underutilisation of advanced practice roles – create further inefficiencies that heighten stress (Buchan et al., 2015). These systemic issues illustrate why workforce planning must be addressed at both macro-policy and organisational levels.

6.1.2 Workload, Burnout and Patient Safety

The link between workload and burnout has been extensively documented. Nurses working in units with high patient-to-nurse ratios are significantly more likely to report emotional exhaustion, job dissatisfaction and intention to leave (Aiken et al., 2002; Vahey et al., 2004). Physicians working more than 60 hours per week report markedly higher rates of burnout and depressive symptoms compared to those with lower workloads (Shanafelt et al., 2012). In a systematic review, Garcia et al. (2020) concluded that workload is among the most consistent predictors of burnout across healthcare professions.

Workload is not only a matter of individual well-being but also a *determinant of patient outcomes*. Higher workloads are associated with increased rates of medical error, lower patient satisfaction and higher mortality (Needleman et al., 2011; Panagioti et al., 2018). For example, a landmark study across 168 hospitals in Pennsylvania showed that each additional patient per nurse was associated with a 7% increase in the likelihood of patient mortality within 30 days of admission (Aiken et al., 2002). These findings underscore that workload management is not a discretionary managerial concern but a patient safety imperative.

6.1.3 Strategies for Workforce Planning

To address these challenges, workforce planning must adopt a *strategic, evidence-based approach* that aligns staffing with patient needs, service demands and long-term demographic trends. Several strategies emerge from the literature.

Evidence strongly supports the introduction of minimum staffing standards (e.g., Buonocore et al., 2025). California's mandated nurse-to-patient ratios, implemented in 2004, were associated with lower mortality and higher job satisfaction (Aiken et al., 2010). Although staffing ratios are not a panacea, they provide an essential safeguard against unsafe workloads.

Beyond fixed ratios, flexible staffing approaches – such as staffing pools, cross-training and the use of predictive analytics – can adapt workforce allocation to fluctuating patient demands (Griffiths et al., 2020). Technology can support real-time workload monitoring, enabling managers to redistribute resources more effectively.

Ensuring the right balance between physicians, nurses and allied health professionals reduces inefficiencies and prevents undue stress on specific groups. Advanced practice nurses, physician assistants and pharmacists can alleviate workload by taking on tasks traditionally confined to physicians (Maier & Aiken, 2016).

Workforce planning must not only recruit but also *retain* staff. Turnover is both costly and destabilising, perpetuating workload stress. Strategies such as mentorship programs, career development opportunities and recognition systems have been shown to improve retention and reduce stress (Shanafelt & Noseworthy, 2017).

Increasingly, organisations are integrating staff well-being into strategic workforce planning frameworks. For example, the United Kingdom's National Health Service (NHS) People Plan explicitly links workforce sustainability to mental health support, flexible scheduling and compassionate leadership (NHS England, 2020). Such approaches recognise that workforce planning is inseparable from workload and well-being management.

6.1.4 Workload Management at the Organisational Level

While macro-level workforce planning sets the stage, *day-to-day workload management* within organisations is equally critical. Leaders play a pivotal role in monitoring and redistributing workload, ensuring equity across teams and responding proactively to staff distress (Cummings et al., 2018). Evidence shows that supportive supervision, participatory scheduling and adequate rest periods significantly reduce stress and improve job satisfaction (Stimpfel et al., 2012).

Technology also offers new opportunities. Electronic rostering systems, workload acuity tools and predictive demand modelling can enhance transparency and fairness in workload distribution (Ball et al., 2014). However, technology must be implemented thoughtfully, as poorly designed systems can add to bureaucratic burden and stress (Shanafelt et al., 2016).

6.2 EVIDENCE-BASED LEADERSHIP PRACTICES FOR STRESS REDUCTION

Leadership is increasingly recognised as a central determinant of healthcare professionals' well-being and a critical lever for reducing occupational stress.

While traditional approaches to stress management often focused on individual coping or organisational policies, recent research demonstrates that the *style and behaviour of leaders* directly shape the psychological climate of healthcare organisations, influencing stress, burnout, resilience and patient outcomes (Cummings et al., 2018; Shanafelt & Noseworthy, 2017). In high-pressure environments such as hospitals and community health services, leadership is not a peripheral concern but a structural factor that either exacerbates or mitigates stress (Riemma, Buonocore et al., 2025).

6.2.1 The Case for Leadership in Stress Mitigation

Healthcare leadership is uniquely challenging because it must balance operational efficiency with compassion, safety and workforce sustainability. Leaders influence stress through multiple mechanisms: by setting expectations, distributing workload, modelling behaviours, creating cultures of support and ensuring recognition (West et al., 2015). Research shows that leadership accounts for a substantial proportion of variance in employee engagement and burnout across healthcare organisations (Sonnentag & Fritz, 2015; Swensen et al., 2016).

For example, transformational leadership (de Gennaro, 2019) – characterised by inspiring vision, individualised consideration and intellectual stimulation – has been consistently linked to lower stress, reduced burnout and higher satisfaction among nurses and physicians (Cummings et al., 2010; Weberg, 2010). In contrast, authoritarian or laissez-faire leadership styles correlate with higher emotional exhaustion, depersonalisation and turnover intentions (Skogstad et al., 2007). These findings underscore the importance of evidence-based leadership practices in mitigating stress and sustaining healthcare systems.

6.2.2 Transformational and Authentic Leadership

Transformational leadership is among the most studied frameworks in healthcare. Cummings et al. (2010), in a systematic review of leadership styles, found that transformational leaders fostered greater nurse empowerment, job satisfaction and organisational commitment. Transformational leaders reduce stress by increasing perceptions of meaning, autonomy and support – factors that buffer the impact of high demands (Laschinger et al., 2012).

Closely related is ***authentic leadership***, which emphasises transparency, ethical behaviour and relational trust. Authentic leaders are perceived as genuine and value-driven, thereby creating climates of psychological safety and reducing stress (Avolio & Gardner, 2005; Wong et al., 2010). Empirical evidence indicates that authentic leadership in healthcare correlates with lower nurse burnout and higher job satisfaction (Laschinger et al., 2015).

6.2.3 Compassionate and Servant Leadership

Recent literature highlights the role of *compassionate leadership* – leaders who listen, empathise and act to alleviate staff suffering – as a particularly powerful approach in healthcare. West et al. (2017) argue that compassionate leadership is not only morally desirable but also instrumental in reducing stress and enhancing patient care. A study in the UK NHS found that units with higher levels of perceived compassionate leadership reported lower staff stress and higher quality-of-care outcomes (West et al., 2020).

Servant leadership, which prioritises the growth and well-being of employees, has also gained attention. Liden et al. (2008) showed that servant leadership predicts higher organisational commitment and lower emotional exhaustion. In healthcare, servant leaders are seen to buffer stress by empowering staff, encouraging collaboration and aligning work with professional values (Neubert et al., 2008).

6.2.4 Distributed and Shared Leadership

While much of the leadership literature focuses on individual leaders, healthcare increasingly benefits from *shared or distributed leadership models*. These approaches recognise that in complex clinical environments, leadership responsibilities are dispersed across professionals and teams rather than concentrated in hierarchical roles (Denis et al., 2012). Shared leadership fosters collective efficacy, mutual support and distributed responsibility, which can reduce stress by preventing overload on individual leaders and promoting resilience across teams (Wang et al., 2014).

In high-stress settings such as emergency departments, shared leadership has been associated with improved communication, lower error rates and better team adaptation under pressure (Künzle et al., 2010). These findings suggest that leadership for stress reduction must be viewed not only as an individual skill but also as an organisational practice embedded in team dynamics.

6.2.5 Evidence-Based Leadership Interventions

Evidence-based practices for leadership in healthcare stress reduction include both individual leader development and systemic organisational initiatives.

Leadership development programs that emphasise emotional intelligence, resilience and supportive communication have shown measurable effects on staff well-being (Clapp-Smith et al., 2009). Training leaders to recognise signs of burnout and respond proactively is now considered an essential component of healthcare management (Shanafelt et al., 2015).

Regular leader rounding – where leaders intentionally check in with staff, listen to concerns and provide feedback – has been linked to reduced stress and increased engagement (Studer, 2003). Visibility and accessibility of leaders during crises, such as COVID-19, were critical in reducing uncertainty and distress (Greenberg et al., 2020; Loia et al., 2022).

Leaders directly influence stress by making equitable workload decisions. Evidence suggests that when leaders are responsive to scheduling concerns, staff report significantly lower stress and higher commitment (Stimpfel et al., 2012).

Recognition is a core element of effort–reward balance (Siegrist, 1996). Leaders who provide timely, sincere recognition reduce perceptions of imbalance and enhance resilience (Brun & Dugas, 2008).

Shanafelt and Noseworthy (2017) proposed nine evidence-based strategies for leaders to reduce physician burnout, including cultivating community at work, aligning values and measuring well-being as a key organisational metric. These practices are increasingly being integrated into healthcare systems worldwide.

6.2.6 Leadership and Psychological Safety

Perhaps the most consistent finding across leadership research is the role of leaders in cultivating *psychological safety* – the shared belief that team members can speak up without fear of reprisal (Edmondson, 2019). Psychological safety is strongly correlated with reduced stress, improved team learning and lower error rates (Nembhard & Edmondson, 2006). Leaders who model openness, admit their own fallibility and encourage questions create environments where stressors are acknowledged and managed collectively rather than silenced.

6.3 PRACTICAL INTERVENTIONS: STAFF SUPPORT, PEER NETWORKS AND DIGITAL TOOLS

While theoretical models and leadership frameworks provide a conceptual lens for understanding stress in healthcare, the ultimate test lies in the implementation of *practical interventions* that address staff well-being directly and sustainably. Across diverse contexts, three domains have gained prominence: structured staff support initiatives, peer-to-peer networks and the use of digital technologies to monitor and mitigate stress. These interventions highlight the need for a pragmatic, evidence-informed approach that complements broader workforce planning and leadership strategies.

Staff support initiatives have long been recognised as vital in preventing burnout and promoting resilience. Programs such as employee assistance services, counselling and structured debriefing sessions provide professionals with a safe outlet to process the emotional toll of healthcare work. Evidence shows that interventions offering confidential psychological support reduce symptoms of anxiety, depression and post-traumatic stress among healthcare workers (Schwappach & Richard, 2018; West et al., 2016). Importantly, staff support must be accessible and normalised. Many professionals hesitate to seek help due to stigma or fear of repercussions, which underscores the importance of leaders explicitly endorsing and participating in such programs (Kinman & Grant, 2020). For example, the 'Schwartz Rounds' model – structured forums for multidisciplinary staff to discuss the emotional and social challenges of care – has been implemented in hospitals across the United Kingdom and the United States, with evaluations showing improvements in empathy, teamwork and staff morale (Maben et al., 2018). These initiatives demonstrate that institutionalising reflective practice and emotional support can directly reduce stress and foster a sense of community.

Alongside formal support structures, *peer networks* represent a powerful, often underutilised, resource in stress mitigation. Peer support programs leverage the shared experiences of healthcare professionals, enabling them to provide emotional, informational and instrumental support to one another. Research has shown that peer networks reduce stigma associated with seeking help, increase resilience and improve retention rates (Hu et al., 2012; Shapiro & Galowitz, 2016). After adverse clinical events, peer support becomes particularly critical. Clinicians involved in medical errors often suffer as 'second victims,' experiencing guilt, shame and trauma (Wu, 2000). Peer support programmes such as the 'forYOU Team' at the University of Missouri have been designed to provide immediate, confidential support to clinicians following such events, with evaluations showing significant reductions in psychological distress and absenteeism (Scott et al., 2010). Moreover, peer mentoring and buddy systems can be used proactively, pairing junior staff with experienced colleagues to navigate role demands and mitigate early stressors. By institutionalising peer networks, healthcare organisations transform solidarity from an informal coping mechanism into a structured form of collective resilience.

Digital tools have emerged as a third frontier of practical intervention, offering innovative means to monitor, predict and alleviate stress in healthcare. Mobile applications for mindfulness, stress tracking and cognitive-behavioural interventions (e.g., Buonocore et al., 2020) have demonstrated efficacy in reducing stress and improving well-being among healthcare professionals (Melnyk et al., 2020; Spadaro & Hunker, 2016). More advanced systems employ real-time data from wearable sensors, electronic health records and scheduling platforms to assess workload and fatigue, enabling managers to intervene before stress escalates into burnout (Rajan et al., 2020). For instance, predictive analytics can be used to identify units with unsafe staffing patterns, while digital dashboards can flag individuals at risk of chronic stress based on work hours and shift patterns. During the COVID-19 pandemic, several hospitals introduced digital platforms that combined mental health resources, peer discussion forums and direct links to professional support, thereby integrating staff support and digital accessibility (Shechter et al., 2020).

Despite their promise, digital tools must be implemented carefully to avoid unintended burdens. Poorly designed systems can exacerbate stress by increasing administrative load or fostering surveillance concerns (Shanafelt et al., 2016). Therefore, successful digital interventions require co-design with frontline staff, ensuring usability, confidentiality and alignment with real needs (Greenhalgh et al., 2017). When thoughtfully deployed, digital tools complement staff support and peer networks by providing scalable, data-driven and personalised approaches to stress reduction.

Taken together, these interventions illustrate a shift from reactive to proactive strategies in managing stress (see Tomo & de Gennaro, 2020). Staff support programmes provide formalised spaces for emotional processing, peer networks embed resilience into professional relationships and digital tools extend the capacity of organisations to monitor and respond dynamically to workload pressures (Riemma, de Gennaro et al., 2025). Crucially, these interventions should not be implemented in isolation but integrated into a broader organisational strategy that prioritises staff well-being as a driver of care quality. When combined with evidence-based leadership and strategic workforce planning, practical interventions form the operational core of stress reduction in healthcare. They ensure that resilience is not left to chance or individual fortitude but embedded in the everyday practices, technologies and cultures of healthcare delivery.

6.4 ORGANISATIONAL LEARNING AND FEEDBACK LOOPS FOR SUSTAINABLE WELL-BEING

A central lesson emerging from both research and practice is that healthcare organisations cannot treat well-being as a static outcome to be achieved once and for all. Rather, staff well-being must be understood as a *dynamic process*, continually shaped by shifting demands, resources and cultural contexts. This recognition calls for the adoption of organisational learning mechanisms and feedback loops that enable healthcare systems to *monitor, reflect and adapt* in real time. Without such adaptive capacities, even well-intentioned interventions risk becoming outdated, symbolic or disconnected from frontline realities.

Organisational learning, as described by Argyris and Schön (1978), involves not only detecting and correcting errors (single-loop learning) but also questioning and revising the underlying norms, policies and assumptions that generate those errors (double-loop learning). Applied to healthcare well-being, this means that organisations should not only adjust work schedules or provide temporary resilience training (single-loop) but also interrogate the deeper structural and cultural drivers of stress, such as chronic understaffing, hierarchical silencing or punitive error cultures (double-loop). More ambitious still, *triple-loop learning* (Flood & Romm, 1996) requires organisations to reflect on how they define 'success' in the first place – reconsidering whether performance metrics that prioritise throughput and cost efficiency over staff well-being and patient safety are truly sustainable.

The interviews with healthcare professionals highlighted how *feedback mechanisms are often weak or absent* in relation to stress and well-being. Many participants expressed scepticism about organisational surveys or audits, describing them as perfunctory exercises with little follow-up. One physician commented: '*We are asked about burnout once a year, but nothing changes. It feels like they collect the data to tick a box, not to act.*' This sentiment aligns with research showing that staff engagement surveys often fail to generate organisational learning when results are not transparently shared or translated into tangible action (Welbourne, 2007).

By contrast, organisations that established *continuous feedback loops* – through regular check-ins, open forums and transparent reporting – were perceived as more responsive and trustworthy. Professionals described how simple practices, such as post-shift debriefings or quarterly well-being reviews, created opportunities for organisational learning and adaptation. These feedback loops not only generated data but also signalled that staff voices were valued, reinforcing psychological safety (Edmondson, 1999). Importantly, effective feedback systems were not one-directional; they enabled *dialogue* rather than mere data collection, fostering a sense of co-ownership of organisational well-being strategies.

The literature on *learning organisations* reinforces this point. Senge (1990) emphasised the importance of 'systems thinking,' where organisations view problems not as isolated events but as interconnected patterns. In healthcare, stress and burnout are often treated symptomatically (e.g., through isolated wellness initiatives) rather than systemically (e.g., redesigning workflows or staffing models). A learning-oriented approach recognises that sustainable well-being requires continuous alignment of *structures, culture and strategy*. This alignment is facilitated by feedback loops that reveal how interventions are working, where gaps persist and how adaptations can be made iteratively.

Another critical element is the use of *data and metrics*. While quantitative indicators such as absenteeism, turnover or patient safety incidents can serve as proxies for staff well-being, they are lagging indicators that often capture problems only after they have escalated. Leading indicators – such as regular pulse surveys, workload tracking or digital monitoring of stress biomarkers (where ethically appropriate) – can provide earlier signals for intervention (Bakker & Demerouti, 2017). Yet data alone is insufficient: without organisational willingness to act, metrics risk becoming performative. Feedback loops must therefore integrate *measurement with action*, ensuring that information translates into timely adjustments.

At the same time, feedback processes must be designed with care to avoid *feedback fatigue*. Professionals in the study voiced frustration at repeated surveys that never led to visible change. As one nurse put it: '*We are tired of being asked how we feel if no one plans to do anything with the answers.*' This underscores the importance of *closing the loop*: organisations must not only collect data but also report back on how feedback has been used to inform decisions. Transparency and accountability are crucial to maintaining trust and sustaining engagement with feedback processes.

Organisational learning for sustainable well-being also requires *distributed responsibility*. While top leaders play a key role in setting the tone and allocating resources, middle managers and frontline leaders are often the most critical actors in translating feedback into practice. Research shows that the impact of leadership on burnout and engagement is particularly strong at the local team level (Shanafelt & Noseworthy, 2017). Empowering these leaders with tools, training and authority to respond to feedback enhances the agility of the system and reduces the gap between strategy and practice.

Ultimately, embedding organisational learning and feedback loops means recognising that *well-being is not a project but a system property*. Just as healthcare organisations monitor infection rates or patient safety indicators on an ongoing basis, they must treat staff well-being as a vital sign of organisational health. This requires institutionalising processes of reflection, dialogue and adaptation – ensuring that interventions remain relevant, staff voices remain central and well-being is woven into the fabric of organisational strategy. As one participant summarised: *'Well-being cannot be managed once a year. It must be part of the daily rhythm of the organization.'*

6.5 DESIGNING SPACES AND RITUALS FOR RECOVERY

Discussions about stress and burnout in healthcare often focus on workload, staffing or leadership. Yet the interviews with professionals and the wider literature make clear that *spaces and rituals* – the physical environments in which care unfolds and the social practices that structure daily life – play a crucial but frequently overlooked role in shaping well-being. Healthcare organisations are not only systems of tasks and hierarchies; they are also lived spaces imbued with routines, rhythms and symbols. These material and cultural dimensions influence whether professionals experience their workplace as exhausting and alienating or as supportive and restorative (de Gennaro & Marino, 2023). Designing spaces and rituals for recovery is therefore a vital component of healthier organisations.

The physical environment of healthcare work exerts direct effects on stress levels. Numerous studies have demonstrated how poor lighting, noise, overcrowding and lack of privacy contribute to fatigue, distraction and burnout (Joseph et al., 2018; Ulrich et al., 2008). Participants in our study frequently emphasised the strain of working in environments that seemed designed for efficiency rather than humanity. One nurse observed: *'There is nowhere to pause, nowhere to catch your breath. Even our break room feels like an afterthought.'* Another professional remarked: *'The walls are grey, the lights are harsh, and you carry the atmosphere with you even when you leave.'* Such testimonies underscore that the materiality of workspaces is not neutral: it shapes the emotional climate of work.

At the same time, research on healthcare architecture highlights the potential of *healing environments* – spaces intentionally designed to reduce stress and promote well-being. Natural light, access to green areas, quiet rooms and ergonomically designed workstations have all been shown to lower stress markers, enhance concentration and support recovery (Mroczek et al., 2005; Ulrich, 1991). The concept of *biophilic design*, which integrates natural elements into built environments, has gained traction as a means of countering the sterile atmospheres of many hospitals (Kellert & Calabrese, 2015). For staff, not only patients, such features can provide micro-moments of respite that replenish emotional resources.

Beyond the physical dimension, *rituals* – the recurrent practices that structure organisational life – also serve as powerful mechanisms of recovery. In the interviews, professionals repeatedly pointed to small, collective practices that helped them decompress: a team sharing coffee after a night shift, a moment of silence before a difficult procedure or humour exchanged during stressful situations. One physician recalled: *'At the end of each week, our team has a short meeting where we share one positive thing that happened. It sounds simple, but it makes a big difference.'* These rituals provide continuity, foster solidarity and signal that well-being is a legitimate part of professional practice.

Organisational scholarship recognises the value of rituals in creating meaning, cohesion and resilience. Trice and Beyer (1984) argue that rituals are symbolic expressions of organisational culture, shaping how members interpret and navigate challenges. In healthcare, rituals of recovery can counterbalance the relentless pace of clinical work by creating intentional pauses. For example, Schwartz Rounds – structured forums for staff to discuss the emotional impact of their work – have been shown to reduce stress, increase empathy and strengthen team cohesion (Goodrich, 2012). These structured rituals complement the informal practices described by participants, suggesting that both institutionalised and spontaneous rituals can enhance collective well-being.

Importantly, spaces and rituals are intertwined. A ritual of debriefing after critical incidents, for instance, requires a dedicated space where staff can gather without interruptions. Similarly, the design of staff rooms influences whether they function as genuine recovery zones or as merely functional extensions of the ward. Too often, participants noted, staff spaces are minimal, noisy or poorly maintained, sending the implicit message that recovery is a low priority. One nurse lamented: *'Patients get gardens and art; we get a windowless room with a vending machine.'* This disparity reflects a deeper organisational blind spot: while patient-centred design has advanced significantly, staff-centred design lags behind, despite clear evidence of its importance for sustainable care.

From a theoretical perspective, these insights align with the Job Demands–Resources (JD-R) model, which emphasises the role of resources in buffering demands (Bakker & Demerouti, 2017). Spaces and rituals function as *recovery resources*, allowing professionals to replenish energy, regulate emotions and reaffirm meaning. Without such resources, high demands accumulate into chronic strain; with them, stress can be metabolised and resilience sustained. Moreover, integrating recovery practices into daily organisational life challenges the notion that well-being is an individual responsibility (e.g., Riemma, de Gennaro et al., 2025). Instead, it positions recovery as a *collective and organisational process*, embedded in design choices and cultural practices.

Designing spaces and rituals for recovery also intersects with broader debates on organisational justice and dignity. When staff are denied adequate spaces for rest or recovery, they perceive not only physical strain but also symbolic disregard. Conversely, when organisations invest in environments and practices that support staff well-being, they communicate respect and recognition. Such signals matter profoundly in professions where identity and meaning are central motivators (Maslach & Leiter, 2016). Providing space and ritual for recovery is thus both a practical intervention and a moral imperative.

The challenge lies in moving from ad hoc initiatives to systematic design. While some hospitals experiment with meditation rooms, quiet pods or regular team debriefings, these remain exceptions rather than norms. To embed recovery into organisational DNA, leaders must treat it as a strategic priority, allocate resources and involve staff in co-designing spaces and rituals that fit their contexts. This participatory approach ensures not only relevance but also ownership, as professionals are more likely to embrace rituals and spaces that reflect their lived realities.

In conclusion, healthcare organisations must recognise that resilience does not arise solely from heroic individuals or supportive teams. It is also cultivated – or undermined – by the spaces in which professionals work and the rituals that shape their days. Designing spaces and rituals for recovery is not a luxury but a necessity for sustainable healthcare. As one participant poignantly put it: *'We give so much to our patients. All we ask is a little space to breathe.'*

6.6 EMPOWERMENT AND CO-DESIGN: GIVING PROFESSIONALS A VOICE[1]

A central tenet of contemporary organisational theory is that sustainable performance and employee well-being cannot be achieved without meaningful participation of workers in shaping the systems in which they operate. This principle has particular resonance in healthcare, where the complexity of work, the interdependence of tasks and the stakes of decision-making require a model of organisation that goes beyond hierarchical control and embraces *empowerment and co-design* as essential strategies. Granting professionals a voice is not only a matter of ethics or symbolic recognition; it is a practical requirement for building resilient and adaptive healthcare systems.

The concept of *employee voice* has received considerable attention in organisational research. Voice is generally defined as the discretionary communication of ideas, concerns or suggestions aimed at improving organisational functioning (Morrison, 2011). Within healthcare, voice is particularly significant because frontline professionals possess critical, experience-based knowledge about clinical workflows, patient needs and organisational constraints. Suppressing or ignoring such knowledge not only undermines staff engagement but can also have direct consequences for patient safety and service quality. The phenomenon of 'organizational silence' (Morrison & Milliken, 2000) describes the collective withholding of input due to fear, futility or cultural barriers – conditions that exacerbate stress, reduce innovation and weaken organisational resilience.

Closely related is the concept of *empowerment*, which has been theorised both structurally and psychologically. Structural empowerment refers to the distribution of power, information and resources that enable individuals to act autonomously and effectively (Kanter, 1977). Psychological empowerment, elaborated by Spreitzer (1995), comprises four dimensions: meaning (the value of work relative to one's ideals), competence (belief in one's capability), self-determination (autonomy in initiating actions) and impact (the extent to which one's actions influence outcomes). Empirical research has consistently linked psychological empowerment to higher engagement, lower burnout and greater organisational commitment (Seibert et al., 2011). In healthcare contexts, empowerment has been shown to foster not only well-being but also patient-centred care and quality improvements (Laschinger et al., 2001).

1 Written by: Ludovica Del Barone, Viviana Colombi Evangelista, Filomena Buonocore, and Davide de Gennaro.

However, empowerment in isolation may remain abstract or symbolic if not translated into *co-design practices* that institutionalise participation. Co-design draws from traditions of participatory design and human-centred innovation, emphasising collaboration between stakeholders in shaping processes, systems and environments (Bate & Robert, 2007). In healthcare, co-design has been applied to redesign care pathways, develop digital tools and improve service delivery, demonstrating tangible benefits for efficiency, safety and staff satisfaction (Donetto et al., 2015). Co-design moves beyond consultation by positioning professionals as active partners rather than passive informants, thereby embedding their expertise into organisational decision-making.

The theoretical foundations of co-design align with broader notions of *organisational justice*. Procedural justice theory emphasises the importance of fair and transparent decision-making processes (Colquitt, 2001; Thibaut & Walker, 1975). When professionals perceive that their voices are heard and that they can influence outcomes, they experience higher levels of trust and legitimacy in organisational decisions. Conversely, exclusion from decision-making fosters perceptions of injustice, which research links to stress, disengagement and turnover intentions (Cropanzano et al., 2007). Empowerment and co-design can thus be understood as mechanisms of organisational justice that directly impact well-being and sustainability.

Another theoretical lens is provided by *sociotechnical systems theory*, which highlights the interdependence of social and technical subsystems within organisations (Trist & Bamforth, 1951). In healthcare, where technological innovations and complex workflows are continuously introduced, the failure to involve professionals in the design of systems often results in misalignments, inefficiencies and stress. Co-design offers a corrective by integrating frontline perspectives into the adaptation of sociotechnical systems, ensuring that new technologies and processes support rather than undermine professional practice.

From the perspective of the *JD-R model* (Bakker & Demerouti, 2017), empowerment and co-design function as critical job resources. By granting autonomy, voice and influence, organisations enable professionals to mobilise personal and collective resources, thereby buffering the impact of high demands. Furthermore, the experience of participation itself enhances motivation and engagement, creating an upward spiral of resources and resilience. The JD-R framework thus provides a useful explanation of why empowerment and co-design are not luxuries but necessities in high-pressure environments such as healthcare (Riemma, Buonocore et al., 2025).

The challenge lies in institutionalising these principles. Without formal structures, empowerment can remain an abstract aspiration, and co-design can devolve into tokenism. Research on participatory practices emphasises the need for *systematic mechanisms* such as joint committees, participatory workshops and digital platforms for feedback (Detert & Burris, 2007; Wilkinson et al., 2020). Equally important is the commitment to 'closing the loop': organisations must demonstrate that staff input has a tangible influence on decisions. Otherwise, participation risks generating cynicism rather than trust.

Critics sometimes argue that empowerment and co-design may slow decision-making or create conflict. However, studies show that structured participation actually enhances organisational adaptability by surfacing diverse perspectives, enabling early identification of problems and fostering collective ownership of solutions (Nembhard & Edmondson, 2006). Particularly in healthcare, where complexity and uncertainty are unavoidable, distributed decision-making is more effective than centralised control. Empowerment and co-design therefore align with contemporary views of *adaptive and relational leadership*, which emphasise collaboration, inclusiveness and responsiveness in dynamic environments (Uhl-Bien et al., 2007).

In sum, empowerment and co-design represent powerful levers for reducing stress and enhancing sustainability in healthcare organisations. They transform professionals from passive recipients of organisational decisions into active co-creators of their work environments. This shift not only enhances individual well-being by increasing autonomy, meaning and fairness but also strengthens organisational resilience by embedding frontline knowledge into continuous improvement processes. Far from being secondary considerations, empowerment and co-design should be seen as central pillars of organisational health strategies – mechanisms that align staff well-being with system performance and that enable healthcare to meet the challenges of an uncertain future.

REFERENCES

Aiken, L. H., Clarke, S. P., Sloane, D. M., Sochalski, J., & Silber, J. H. (2002). Hospital nurse staffing and patient mortality, nurse burnout, and job dissatisfaction. *JAMA*, *288*(16), 1987–1993.

Aiken, L. H., Sermeus, W., Van den Heede, K., Sloane, D. M., Busse, R., McKee, M., Bruyneel, L., Rafferty, A. M., Griffiths, P., Moreno-Casbas, M. T., Tishelman, C., Scott, A., Brzostek, T., Kinnunen, J., Schwendimann, R., Heinen, M., Zikos, D., Sjetne, I. S., Smith, H. L., & Kutney-Lee, A. (2012). Patient safety, satisfaction, and quality of hospital care: Cross sectional surveys of nurses and patients in 12 countries in Europe and the United States. *BMJ*, *344*, e1717.

Aiken, L. H., Sloane, D. M., Cimiotti, J. P., Clarke, S. P., Flynn, L., Seago, J. A., Spetz, J., & Smith, H. L. (2010). Implications of the California nurse staffing mandate for other states. *Health Services Research*, *45*(4), 904–921.

Argyris, C., & Schön, D. A. (1978). *Organizational learning: A theory of action perspective*. Addison-Wesley.

Avolio, B. J., & Gardner, W. L. (2005). Authentic leadership development: Getting to the root of positive forms of leadership. *The Leadership Quarterly*, *16*(3), 315–338.

Bakker, A. B., & Demerouti, E. (2017). Job demands–resources theory: Taking stock and looking forward. *Journal of Occupational Health Psychology*, *22*(3), 273–285.

Ball, J. E., Murrells, T., Rafferty, A. M., Morrow, E., & Griffiths, P. (2014). 'Care left undone' during nursing shifts: Associations with workload and perceived quality of care. *BMJ Quality and Safety*, *23*(2), 116–125.

Bate, P., & Robert, G. (2007). *Bringing user experience to healthcare improvement: The concepts, methods and practices of experience-based design*. Radcliffe Publishing.

Brun, J. P., & Dugas, N. (2008). An analysis of employee recognition: Perspectives on human resources practices. *International Journal of Human Resource Management*, *19*(4), 716–730.

Buchan, J., Duffield, C., & Jordan, A. (2015). 'Solving' nursing shortages: Do we need a new agenda? *Journal of Nursing Management*, *23*(5), 543–545.

Buonocore, F., de Gennaro, D., & Del Barone, L. (2025). Ethical and organizational dynamics of non-standard work in public administration: Challenges and opportunities in the digital era. *Personnel Review. ahead-of-print*. https://doi.org/10.1108/PR-05-2024-0506

Buonocore, F., de Gennaro, D., Russo, M., & Salvatore, D. (2020). Cognitive job crafting: A possible response to increasing job insecurity and declining professional prestige. *Human Resource Management Journal*, *30* (2), 244–259. ISSN: 1748-8583. https://doi.org/10.1111/1748-8583.12270

Campbell, J., Buchan, J., Cometto, G., David, B., Dussault, G., Fogstad, H., Fronteira, I., Lozano, R., Nyonator, F., Pablos-Mendez, A., Quain, E.,

Starrs, A., & Tangcharoensathien, V. (2013). Human resources for health and universal health coverage: Fostering equity and effective coverage. *Bulletin of the World Health Organization*, *91*(11), 853–863.

Clapp-Smith, R., Vogelgesang, G. R., & Avey, J. B. (2009). Authentic leadership and positive psychological capital: The mediating role of trust at the group level of analysis. *Journal of Leadership & Organizational Studies*, *15*(3), 227–240.

Colquitt, J. A. (2001). On the dimensionality of organizational justice: A construct validation of a measure. *Journal of Applied Psychology*, *86*(3), 386–400.

Cropanzano, R., Bowen, D. E., & Gilliland, S. W. (2007). The management of organizational justice. *Academy of Management Perspectives*, *21*(4), 34–48.

Cummings, G. G., MacGregor, T., Davey, M., Lee, H., Wong, C. A., Lo, E., Muise, M., & Stafford, E. (2010). Leadership styles and outcome patterns for the nursing workforce and work environment: A systematic review. *International Journal of Nursing Studies*, *47*(3), 363–385.

Cummings, G. G., Tate, K., Lee, S., Wong, C. A., Paananen, T., Micaroni, S. P., & Chatterjee, G. E. (2018). Leadership styles and outcome patterns for the nursing workforce and work environment: A systematic review. *International Journal of Nursing Studies*, *85*, 19–60.

Dall'Ora, C., Griffiths, P., Ball, J., Simon, M., & Aiken, L. H. (2015). Association of 12 h shifts and nurses' job satisfaction, burnout and intention to leave: Findings from a cross-sectional study of 12 European countries. *BMJ Open*, *5*(9), e008331.

de Gennaro, D. (2019). Transformational leadership for public service motivation. *Journal of Economic and Administrative Sciences*, *35*(1), 5–15. ISSN: 1026-4116. https://doi.org/10.1108/JEAS-06-2018-0075

de Gennaro, D., & Marino, M. (2023). *Cross-cultural undergraduate internships: A toolkit for empowering the next generation*. Emerald Publishing Limited. ISBN: 978-1-80455-357-2, eISBN: 978-1-80455-356-5. https://doi.org/10.1108/9781804553565

Denis, J. L., Langley, A., & Sergi, V. (2012). Leadership in the plural. *The Academy of Management Annals*, *6*(1), 211–283.

Detert, J. R., & Burris, E. R. (2007). Leadership behavior and employee voice: Is the door really open? *Academy of Management Journal*, *50*(4), 869–884.

Donetto, S., Pierri, P., Tsianakas, V., & Robert, G. (2015). Experience-based co-design and healthcare improvement: Realizing participatory design in the public sector. *The Design Journal*, *18*(2), 227–248.

Edmondson, A. C. (1999). Psychological safety and learning behavior in work teams. *Administrative Science Quarterly*, *44*(2), 350–383.

Edmondson, A. C. (2019). *The fearless organization: Creating psychological safety in the workplace for learning, innovation, and growth*. Wiley.

Flood, R. L., & Romm, N. R. A. (1996). *Diversity management: Triple loop learning*. Wiley.

Garcia, C. L., Abreu, L. C., Ramos, J. L. S., Castro, C. F. D., Smiderle, F. R. N., Santos, J. A. D., & Bezerra, I. M. P. (2020). Influence of burnout on patient safety: Systematic review and meta-analysis. *Medicina*, *55*(9).

Goodrich, J. (2012). Supporting hospital staff to provide compassionate care: Do Schwartz Center Rounds work in English hospitals? *Journal of the Royal Society of Medicine*, *105*(3), 117–122.

Greenberg, N., Docherty, M., Gnanapragasam, S., & Wessely, S. (2020). Managing mental health challenges faced by healthcare workers during COVID-19. *BMJ*, *368*, m1211.

Greenhalgh, T., Wherton, J., Papoutsi, C., Lynch, J., & Hughes, G. (2017). Beyond adoption: A new framework for theorizing and evaluating nonadoption, abandonment, and challenges to the scale-up, spread, and sustainability of health and care technologies. *Journal of Medical Internet Research*, *19*(11), e367.

Griffiths, P., Maruotti, A., Recio Saucedo, A., Redfern, O. C., Ball, J. E., Briggs, J., Dall'Ora, C., Schmidt, P. E., & Smith, G. B. (2020). Nurse staffing, nursing assistants and hospital mortality: Retrospective longitudinal cohort study. *BMJ Quality & Safety*, *28*(8), 609–617.

Hu, Y. Y., Fix, M. L., Hevelone, N. D., Lipsitz, S. R., Greenberg, C. C., & Shapiro, J. (2012). Physicians' needs in coping with emotional stressors: The case for peer support. *Archives of Surgery*, *147*(3), 212–217.

Joseph, A., Quan, X., Keller, A., & Taylor, E. (2018). Designing for safety: Evidence-based design and healthcare-associated infections. *HERD: Health Environments Research & Design Journal*, *11*(1), 11–26.

Kanter, R. M. (1977). *Men and women of the corporation*. Basic Books.

Kellert, S. R., & Calabrese, E. (2015). *The practice of biophilic design*. Terrapin Bright Green.

Kinman, G., & Grant, L. (2020). Presenteeism during the COVID-19 pandemic: Risks and solutions. *Occupational Medicine*, *70*(5), 243–244.

Künzle, B., Zala-Mezö, E., & Grote, G. (2010). Leadership in anaesthesia teams: The most effective leadership is shared. *Anesthesia & Analgesia*, *111* (4), 932–937.

Laschinger, H. K. S., Finegan, J., Shamian, J., & Wilk, P. (2001). Impact of structural and psychological empowerment on job strain in nursing work settings: Expanding Kanter's model. *The Journal of Nursing Administration*, *31*(5), 260–272.

Laschinger, H. K. S., Wong, C. A., Cummings, G. G., & Grau, A. L. (2015). Resonant leadership and workplace empowerment: The value of positive organizational cultures in reducing burnout in nursing. *International Journal of Nursing Studies*, *52*(12), 1785–1796.

Laschinger, H. K. S., Wong, C. A., & Grau, A. L. (2012). Authentic leadership, empowerment, and burnout: A comparison in new graduates and experienced nurses. *Journal of Nursing Management*, *20*(3), 522–532.

Liden, R. C., Wayne, S. J., Zhao, H., & Henderson, D. (2008). Servant leadership: Development of a multidimensional measure and multi-level assessment. *The Leadership Quarterly*, *19*(2), 161–177.

Loia, F., de Gennaro, D., & Adinolfi, P. (2022). Managerial hubristic-behavioral strategy: How to cope with chaotic and uncertain contexts. *Management Research Review*, *45*(9), 1137–1154. ISSN: 2040-8269. https://doi.org/10.1108/MRR-11-2021-0811

Maben, J., Bridges, J., Adams, M., Peccei, R., Murrells, T., & Robert, G. (2018). Recognising and rewarding compassionate care: Exploring the implications of the Francis report for nurse education and practice. *Journal of Nursing Management*, *26*(4).

Maier, C. B., & Aiken, L. H. (2016). Task shifting from physicians to nurses in primary care in 39 countries: A cross-country comparative study. *European Journal of Public Health*, 26(6), 927–934.

Maslach, C., & Leiter, M. P. (2016). Burnout: A multidimensional perspective. In C. L. Cooper & P. J. Dewe (Eds.), *Stress: Concepts, cognition, emotion, and behavior* (pp. 351–357). Academic Press.

Melnyk, B. M., Kelly, S. A., Stephens, J., Dhakal, K., McGovern, C., Tucker, S., Hoying, J., McCarthy, M., Spurlock, E., & Bird, S. B. (2020). Interventions to improve mental health, well-being, physical health, and lifestyle behaviors in physicians and nurses: A systematic review. *American Journal of Health Promotion*, *34*(8), 929–941.

Morrison, E. W. (2011). Employee voice behavior: Integration and directions for future research. *The Academy of Management Annals*, *5*(1), 373–412.

Morrison, E. W., & Milliken, F. J. (2000). Organizational silence: A barrier to change and development in a pluralistic world. *Academy of Management Review*, *25*(4), 706–725.

Mroczek, J., Mikitarian, G., Vieira, E., & Rotthoff, R. (2005). Hospital design and staff perceptions: An exploratory analysis. *HERD: Health Environments Research & Design Journal*, *1*(1), 71–85.

Needleman, J., Buerhaus, P., Pankratz, S., Leibson, C. L., Stevens, S. R., & Harris, M. (2011). Nurse staffing and inpatient hospital mortality. *New England Journal of Medicine*, *364*(11), 1037–1045.

Nembhard, I. M., & Edmondson, A. C. (2006). Making it safe: The effects of leader inclusiveness and professional status on psychological safety and improvement efforts in health care teams. *Journal of Organizational Behavior*, 27(7), 941–966.

Neubert, M. J., Kacmar, K. M., Carlson, D. S., Chonko, L. B., & Roberts, J. A. (2008). Regulatory focus as a mediator of the influence of initiating structure and servant leadership on employee behavior. *Journal of Applied Psychology*, *93*(6), 1220–1233.

NHS England. (2020). *We are the NHS: People plan for 2020/21 – action for us all*. NHS England.

Panagioti, M., Geraghty, K., Johnson, J., Zhou, A., Panagopoulou, E., Chew-Graham, C., Peters, D., Hodkinson, A., Riley, R., & Esmail, A.

(2018). Association between physician burnout and patient safety, professionalism, and patient satisfaction: A systematic review and meta-analysis. *JAMA Internal Medicine, 178*(10), 1317–1330.

Rajan, S., Thirunavukkarasu, A., & Seymour, N. (2020). Wearable devices and healthcare: Data-driven approaches to stress and fatigue. *Journal of Medical Systems, 44*(7), 125.

Riemma, F., Buonocore, F., & de Gennaro, D. (2025). Coping with pressure: Stress management and organizational support in healthcare settings. *Personnel Review. ahead-of-print.* https://doi.org/10.1108/PR-04-2025-0387

Riemma, F., de Gennaro, D., Buonocore, F., & Annosi, M. C. (2025). Plural masculinities at work: Generational cohorts, organizational culture, and men's work-life choices. *Career Development International. ahead-of-print.* https://doi.org/10.1108/CDI-11-2024-0501

Schwappach, D. L. B., & Richard, A. (2018). Speak up-related climate and its association with healthcare workers' speaking up and withholding voice behaviours: A cross-sectional survey in Switzerland. *BMJ Open, 8*(4), e020586.

Scott, S. D., Hirschinger, L. E., Cox, K. R., McCoig, M., Brandt, J., & Hall, L. W. (2010). The natural history of recovery for the healthcare provider "second victim" after adverse patient events. *Quality and Safety in Health Care, 18*(5), 325–330.

Seibert, S. E., Wang, G., & Courtright, S. H. (2011). Antecedents and consequences of psychological and team empowerment in organizations: A meta-analytic review. *Journal of Applied Psychology, 96*(5), 981–1003.

Senge, P. M. (1990). *The fifth discipline: The art and practice of the learning organization.* Doubleday.

Shanafelt, T. D., Hasan, O., Dyrbye, L. N., Sinsky, C., Satele, D., Sloan, J., & West, C. P. (2015). Changes in burnout and satisfaction with work-life balance in physicians and the general US working population between 2011 and 2014. *Mayo Clinic Proceedings, 90*(12), 1600–1613.

Shanafelt, T. D., Boone, S., Tan, L., Dyrbye, L. N., Sotile, W., Satele, D., West, C. P., Sloan, J., & Oreskovich, M. R. (2012). Burnout and satisfaction with work-life balance among US physicians relative to the general US population. *Archives of Internal Medicine, 172*(18), 1377–1385.

Shanafelt, T. D., Dyrbye, L. N., & West, C. P. (2016). Addressing physician burnout: The way forward. *JAMA, 317*(9), 901–902.

Shanafelt, T. D., & Noseworthy, J. H. (2017). Executive leadership and physician well-being: Nine organizational strategies to promote engagement and reduce burnout. *Mayo Clinic Proceedings*, 92(1), 129–146.

Shapiro, J., & Galowitz, P. (2016). Peer support for clinicians: A programmatic approach. *Academic Medicine, 91*(9), 1200–1204.

Shechter, A., Diaz, F., Moise, N., Anstey, D. E., Ye, S., Agarwal, S., Birk, J. L., Brodie, D., Cannone, D. E., Chang, B., Claassen, J., Cornelius, T., Derby, L., Dong, M., Givens, R. C., Hochman, B., Homma, S., Kronish, I. M., Lee, S. A., & Abdalla, M. (2020). Psychological distress, coping behaviors, and preferences for support among New York healthcare workers during the COVID-19 pandemic. *General Hospital Psychiatry*, 66, 1–8.

Siegrist, J. (1996). Adverse health effects of high-effort/low-reward conditions. *Journal of Occupational Health Psychology, 1*(1), 27–41.

Skogstad, A., Einarsen, S., Torsheim, T., Aasland, M. S., & Hetland, H. (2007). The destructiveness of laissez-faire leadership behavior. *Journal of Occupational Health Psychology, 12*(1), 80–92.

Sonnentag, S., & Fritz, C. (2015). Recovery from job stress: The stressor–detachment model as an integrative framework. *Journal of Organizational Behavior, 36*(S1), S72–S103.

Spadaro, K. C., & Hunker, D. F. (2016). Exploring the effects of an online asynchronous mindfulness meditation intervention with nursing students on stress, mood, and cognition: A descriptive study. *Nurse Education Today, 39*, 163–169.

Spreitzer, G. M. (1995). Psychological empowerment in the workplace: Dimensions, measurement, and validation. *Academy of Management Journal, 38*(5), 1442–1465.

Stimpfel, A. W., Sloane, D. M., & Aiken, L. H. (2012). The longer the shifts for hospital nurses, the higher the levels of burnout and patient dissatisfaction. *Health Affairs, 31*(11), 2501–2509.

Studer, Q. (2003). *Hardwiring excellence: Purpose, worthwhile work, making a difference*. Fire Starter Publishing.

Swensen, S., Kabcenell, A., & Shanafelt, T. (2016). Physician–organization collaboration reduces physician burnout and promotes engagement: The

Mayo Clinic experience. *Journal of Healthcare Management, 61*(2), 105–127.

Thibaut, J., & Walker, L. (1975). *Procedural justice: A psychological analysis*. Erlbaum.

Tomo, A., & de Gennaro, D. (2020). Accountants' behavioural reactions to external threats: The mediating role of proactive personality in the goal orientation process. *Meditari Accountancy Research, 29*(6), 1337–1353. ISSN: 2049-372X. https://doi.org/10.1108/MEDAR-04-2020-0843

Trice, H. M., & Beyer, J. M. (1984). Studying organizational cultures through rites and ceremonials. *Academy of Management Review, 9*(4), 653–669.

Trist, E. L., & Bamforth, K. W. (1951). Some social and psychological consequences of the longwall method of coal-getting. *Human Relations, 4*(1), 3–38.

Uhl-Bien, M., Marion, R., & McKelvey, B. (2007). Complexity leadership theory: Shifting leadership from the industrial age to the knowledge era. *The Leadership Quarterly, 18*(4), 298–318.

Ulrich, R. S. (1991). Effects of interior design on wellness: Theory and recent scientific research. *Journal of Health Care Interior Design, 3*(1), 97–109.

Ulrich, R. S., Zimring, C., Zhu, X., DuBose, J., Seo, H.-B., Choi, Y.-S., Quan, X., & Joseph, A. (2008). A review of the research literature on evidence-based healthcare design. *HERD: Health Environments Research & Design Journal, 1*(3), 61–125.

Vahey, D. C., Aiken, L. H., Sloane, D. M., Clarke, S. P., & Vargas, D. (2004). Nurse burnout and patient satisfaction. *Medical Care, 42*(2), II57–II66.

Wang, D., Waldman, D. A., & Zhang, Z. (2014). A meta-analysis of shared leadership and team effectiveness. *Journal of Applied Psychology, 99*(2), 181–198.

Weberg, D. (2010). Transformational leadership and staff retention: An evidence review with implications for healthcare systems. *Nursing Administration Quarterly, 34*(3), 246–258.

Welbourne, T. M. (2007). Employee surveys: Why do workers distrust them? *Human Resource Management, 46*(3), 315–333.

West, M., Armit, K., Loewenthal, L., Eckert, R., West, T., & Lee, A. (2015). *Leadership and leadership development in health care: The evidence base.* Faculty of Medical Leadership and Management.

West, M., Bailey, S., & Williams, E. (2020). *The courage of compassion: Supporting nurses and midwives to deliver high-quality care.* The King's Fund.

West, C. P., Dyrbye, L. N., Erwin, P. J., & Shanafelt, T. D. (2016). Interventions to prevent and reduce physician burnout: A systematic review and meta-analysis. *The Lancet, 388*(10057), 2272–2281.

West, M., Eckert, R., Collins, B., & Chowla, R. (2017). *Caring to change: How compassionate leadership can stimulate innovation in health care.* The King's Fund.

Wilkinson, A., Donaghey, J., Dundon, T., & Freeman, R. (2020). *Handbook of research on employee voice.* Edward Elgar Publishing.

Wong, C. A., Cummings, G. G., & Ducharme, L. (2010). The relationship between nursing leadership and patient outcomes: A systematic review. *Journal of Nursing Management, 18*(8), 889–900.

World Health Organization. (2016). *Global strategy on human resources for health: Workforce 2030.* WHO.

World Health Organization. (2020). *State of the World's nursing 2020: Investing in education, jobs and leadership.* WHO.

Wu, A. W. (2000). Medical error: The second victim. *BMJ, 320*(7237), 726–727.

Part IV

FROM CRISIS TO SUSTAINABILITY

INTRODUCTION

The preceding chapters have demonstrated that stress in healthcare is not an episodic challenge to be managed temporarily but a structural condition embedded in the very fabric of modern healthcare systems. From the acute crises of the COVID-19 pandemic to the chronic challenges of workforce shortages, organisational inefficiencies and moral distress, stress has proven to be both enduring and multifaceted. We have also seen how traditional theories, organisational practices and leadership frameworks provide essential insights, yet often require adaptation to account for the unique realities of healthcare. In Part III, we argued that stress cannot be resolved solely at the level of the individual professional: it is a systemic issue that demands systemic solutions.

Part IV – From Crisis to Sustainability takes this argument forward by focusing on the conditions under which healthcare systems can move from short-term, crisis-driven responses to long-term strategies for sustainability and resilience. Sustainability here is not limited to financial or operational viability; it encompasses the capacity of healthcare organisations to maintain *staff well-being, high-quality patient care and organisational adaptability* over time. In other words, sustainability is about building healthcare systems that do not simply endure stress but actively transform it into a catalyst for innovation, improvement and resilience.

This requires a dual lens. On the one hand, healthcare organisations must continue to address immediate stressors – workload, staffing, emotional demands – through evidence-based interventions. On the other hand, they must engage in *structural and cultural reforms* that create environments where stress is not only reduced but also managed in ways that support learning, collaboration and professional growth. The transition from crisis to sustainability therefore involves reimagining stress management as part of a broader strategy of organisational development and system-wide transformation.

The chapters in this part examine how such a transition can be realised. Chapter 7 explores the challenge of bridging theory and practice, showing how models of stress and resilience can inform real-world interventions without oversimplifying the complexities of healthcare work. Chapter 8 reflects on policy, leadership and systemic change, asking what structural conditions are necessary to embed sustainability at the level of entire healthcare systems. Finally, the conclusion synthesises these insights, highlighting pathways for healthcare organisations to move beyond reactive coping and towards proactive, integrated strategies that align workforce well-being with the long-term goals of patient care and organisational resilience.

In setting the stage for these discussions, it is worth emphasising that sustainability is not a static end state but an ongoing process of adaptation. Healthcare is – and will remain – a high-pressure environment. What distinguishes sustainable systems from fragile ones is not the absence of stress but the ability to channel stress constructively, prevent its most harmful effects and transform challenges into opportunities for innovation and improvement. This is the ultimate promise of moving from crisis to sustainability: creating healthcare systems that protect their workers, serve their patients and endure with resilience in the face of uncertainty.

7

BRIDGING THEORY AND PRACTICE

ABSTRACT

This chapter bridges theory and practice by demonstrating that healthcare professionals' well-being and the quality of patient care are intrinsically interdependent rather than competing priorities. Drawing on a robust body of empirical evidence, this chapter shows how staff burnout, moral distress and compassion fatigue are directly associated with medical errors, reduced patient satisfaction and compromised safety, while supportive organisational conditions simultaneously enhance workforce well-being and care quality. Well-being and patient outcomes are thus conceptualised as two sides of the same systemic dynamic.

This chapter explores the organisational mechanisms that mediate this relationship, including staffing levels, workload, leadership, team climate and organisational culture. Using the Job Demands–Resources framework, it illustrates how excessive demands and insufficient resources generate a downward spiral of burnout and declining care quality, whereas supportive leadership, psychological safety and recognition foster engagement, learning and safer care. The analysis highlights the moral dimension of this interdependence, emphasising how moral distress undermines both professional integrity and patient outcomes.

Moving beyond diagnosis, this chapter argues for the strategic alignment of leadership practices, policy frameworks and workforce strategies. Fragmentation across these domains perpetuates stress and inefficiency, while alignment creates virtuous cycles of resilience, retention and quality improvement. Drawing on examples from integrated health systems, this chapter demonstrates how sustained leadership commitment, supportive policy environments and robust workforce planning can jointly reduce stress and enhance performance.

Keywords: Staff well-being; patient safety; moral distress; healthcare sustainability; organisational resilience

7.1 WHY WELL-BEING AND PATIENT CARE ARE TWO SIDES OF THE SAME COIN

For decades, healthcare systems have treated the well-being of staff and the quality of patient care as if they were separate priorities, often placing them in implicit competition for scarce resources. Investments in patient safety, clinical innovation and efficiency have frequently been pursued at the expense of workforce well-being, while initiatives aimed at supporting staff have sometimes been dismissed as secondary to the 'real' work of delivering care. Yet a growing body of evidence demonstrates that this dichotomy is fundamentally false. In reality, the well-being of healthcare professionals and the quality of patient care are not competing goals but *two sides of the same coin* – interdependent, mutually reinforcing and essential to the sustainability of healthcare systems (West et al., 2020).

7.1.1 The Evidence Linking Staff Well-Being and Patient Outcomes

A robust empirical literature confirms the direct and indirect links between staff well-being and patient outcomes. Burnout among physicians and nurses is strongly associated with higher rates of medical error, reduced quality of care, lower patient satisfaction and even increased patient mortality (Panagioti et al., 2018; Tawfik et al., 2019). For instance, a large cross-sectional study by Hall et al. (2016) found that staff burnout was significantly correlated with patient safety incidents across multiple clinical settings. Similarly, Aiken et al. (2002) demonstrated that hospitals with higher nurse-to-patient ratios had not only higher levels of nurse burnout but also significantly higher patient mortality rates. These findings underscore that the quality of care cannot be insulated from the conditions under which it is delivered.

Beyond clinical outcomes, patient experience is closely tied to staff well-being. Healthcare professionals who are emotionally exhausted or depersonalised often struggle to maintain empathy and effective communication, leading to diminished trust and satisfaction (West et al., 2018a). A systematic review by Dyrbye et al. (2020) concluded that physician burnout undermines the patient–physician relationship, increasing the risk of miscommunication, lower adherence to treatment and patient dissatisfaction. Compassion fatigue, a common consequence of chronic stress, has been shown to erode the therapeutic alliance that is central to healing (Figley, 2002; Peters, 2018). Thus, the erosion of well-being among staff directly translates into an erosion of care quality and patient experience.

7.1.2 The Moral and Professional Nexus

The relationship between well-being and patient care is not merely instrumental but deeply moral. Healthcare professionals often enter the field motivated by altruism, compassion and a desire to serve. When systemic conditions undermine their ability to provide high-quality care, professionals experience *moral distress* – the psychological disequilibrium that arises when they know the right thing to do but are constrained from doing it (Epstein & Hamric, 2009; Jameton, 1984). Moral distress contributes to burnout, attrition and a loss of professional identity, but it also compromises patient care by normalising unsafe or substandard practices. Rushton (2018) and Del Barone et al. (2025) argue that moral resilience – the ability to sustain or restore integrity in response to ethical challenges – is as critical to patient safety as technical competence (see also Gagliarducci & de Gennaro, 2020). In this sense, protecting staff well-being is also about safeguarding the moral fabric of care.

7.1.3 The Organisational Mechanisms of Interdependence

The interdependence of well-being and patient care is mediated through organisational mechanisms that simultaneously affect staff and patients. Staffing levels, workload, leadership and culture create the conditions in which both professionals and patients thrive – or suffer. The Job Demands–Resources (JD-R) model (Bakker & Demerouti, 2007) provides a useful framework for understanding these dynamics: when demands are excessive and resources insufficient, staff experience burnout, which in turn diminishes engagement, teamwork and ultimately care quality. Conversely, when organisations invest in resources – such as supportive leadership, recognition and autonomy – staff engagement rises, leading to improved patient outcomes (Schaufeli & Bakker, 2004).

One organisational mechanism is *team climate*. Edmondson (2019) demonstrates that psychological safety – the shared belief that team members can speak up without fear of reprisal – is crucial for both staff well-being and patient safety. Teams with high psychological safety not only report fewer errors but also experience lower stress and higher morale (Nembhard & Edmondson, 2006). Another mechanism is leadership: compassionate and transformational leadership styles (de Gennaro, 2019) reduce staff burnout while simultaneously improving patient satisfaction and safety metrics (Cummings et al., 2018; West et al., 2017). These findings make clear that organisations cannot meaningfully pursue patient safety agendas without simultaneously addressing workforce well-being.

7.1.4 Economic and Strategic Implications

The link between staff well-being and patient care is also reflected in economic terms. Burnout and stress among healthcare professionals drive turnover, absenteeism and presenteeism, leading to significant financial costs for organisations. Replacing a single physician who leaves due to burnout costs an estimated $250,000–$500,000 in recruitment and lost productivity (Han et al., 2019). Nurse turnover similarly destabilises staffing levels and increases reliance on costly temporary staff (Dall'Ora et al., 2020). These disruptions directly affect continuity of care, teamwork and patient outcomes. Conversely, organisations that invest in well-being interventions not only reduce burnout but also achieve better retention, more consistent staffing and improved patient safety outcomes (West et al., 2020). From a strategic perspective, aligning well-being and patient care is not just ethically compelling but also financially prudent.

7.1.5 Moving Beyond the False Dichotomy

Why, then, has the false dichotomy between staff well-being and patient care persisted? One reason is the tendency to treat staff well-being as a private or individual matter, rather than a systemic concern. Interventions have often focused narrowly on teaching individuals to cope better – through mindfulness, resilience training or stress management workshops – without addressing structural stressors such as staffing shortages or excessive administrative burden (de Gennaro & Marino, 2024; Kinman & Grant, 2020; West et al., 2018b). While individual interventions can be valuable, they are insufficient if organisational conditions remain toxic. Healthcare thus offers a crucial insight for stress theory: *well-being and patient care cannot be disentangled because they are mediated by the same systemic conditions.*

Another reason is the short-termism of healthcare policy and management. Under pressure to meet immediate performance targets, organisations may prioritise throughput and efficiency at the expense of workforce sustainability (Riemma et al., 2025). Yet the evidence shows that this is a false economy. Short-term gains achieved by overloading staff ultimately lead to long-term costs in the form of burnout, turnover and compromised patient outcomes (Shanafelt et al., 2017). By contrast, organisations that take a long-term perspective – investing in staff support, leadership development and safe staffing – achieve both higher staff satisfaction and superior patient outcomes.

7.2 ALIGNING LEADERSHIP, POLICY AND WORKFORCE STRATEGIES

If well-being and patient care are indeed two sides of the same coin, then the challenge for healthcare organisations is to align leadership practices, policy frameworks and workforce strategies into a coherent and mutually reinforcing system. Too often, these domains operate in silos: leadership initiatives are launched without integration into policy priorities; workforce plans are developed without sustained leadership buy-in; and policies are implemented with little attention to their real impact on frontline staff. The result is fragmentation, inefficiency and, ultimately, a widening gap between ambitious strategic goals and the lived experience of healthcare professionals. Moving towards sustainable healthcare requires recognising that leadership, policy and workforce strategies are interdependent elements of a single ecosystem that must be aligned if stress is to be reduced and resilience enhanced.

The first dimension of this alignment involves *leadership commitment.* Evidence shows that leadership engagement at the highest levels is a critical determinant of whether well-being and workforce strategies are successful (Shanafelt & Noseworthy, 2017). Leaders who prioritise staff well-being in organisational vision and resource allocation signal that these issues are not peripheral but central to quality and sustainability. Without this commitment, workforce initiatives often remain underfunded or symbolic, producing little tangible impact. Moreover, alignment requires not only formal endorsement but also consistent role modelling: leaders must embody the values of compassion, integrity and openness that they expect from their teams (West et al., 2017). Studies in both nursing and medicine demonstrate that when leaders actively demonstrate care for staff – through visible presence, responsiveness to concerns and equitable workload decisions – burnout decreases and engagement increases (Cummings et al., 2018; Swensen et al., 2016).

The second dimension is *policy integration*. National and regional policies shape the structural environment of healthcare organisations, from staffing ratios and funding mechanisms to professional development and regulatory standards. Policies that prioritise throughput, cost-cutting, or bureaucratic efficiency may inadvertently undermine professional autonomy and staff well-being (Dyrbye et al., 2020). Conversely, policies that explicitly link workforce well-being to care quality – such as the National Health Service (NHS) People Plan in England (NHS England, 2020) – provide a framework for organisations to align their strategies with national priorities. Research suggests that policy environments that mandate safe staffing levels, provide protected time for training and support flexible working arrangements are associated with lower burnout and improved retention (Aiken et al., 2012; Griffiths et al., 2020). Importantly, policy must also address the ethical dimensions of care: guidelines and regulations that reduce moral distress by clarifying roles, expectations and support for ethical decision-making can reduce stress across professions (Epstein & Hamric, 2009; Rushton, 2018).

The third dimension is *workforce strategy*, which operationalises leadership and policy commitments into day-to-day practices. Workforce planning, workload management, recruitment and retention strategies are not merely technical issues but central determinants of well-being and patient outcomes (Aiken et al., 2002; Buchan et al., 2015). Aligning workforce strategies with leadership and policy requires a long-term perspective: ensuring adequate staffing pipelines through investment in education, balancing skill mix to maximise efficiency and reduce stress, and embedding recognition and career development opportunities into human resource policies. In this sense, workforce strategy becomes the bridge between policy aspirations and frontline realities. Without adequate workforce planning, even the most compassionate leadership and supportive policies cannot be translated into sustainable practice.

When leadership, policy and workforce strategies are misaligned, healthcare systems experience a vicious cycle. For example, a policy mandating efficiency targets without adequate workforce planning can lead leaders to push staff beyond sustainable limits, exacerbating burnout and attrition (Shanafelt et al., 2017). Conversely, when these domains are aligned, a virtuous cycle emerges: supportive policies enable effective workforce strategies, which are championed and reinforced by leadership, resulting in reduced stress, improved care and greater organisational resilience (Del Barone et al., 2025).

One of the most compelling illustrations of alignment comes from integrated health systems that have explicitly linked workforce well-being to strategic goals. The Mayo Clinic, for instance, developed a comprehensive programme in which leadership accountability, organisational policy and workforce development were all oriented towards reducing burnout and promoting engagement (Swensen et al., 2016). The programme included regular measurement of well-being, leadership training and structural changes to reduce clerical burden, demonstrating measurable improvements in physician engagement and patient care quality. Similarly, in the United Kingdom, the implementation of the Francis Report recommendations emphasised compassionate leadership, national policy changes and workforce investment as mutually reinforcing strategies for improving both staff experience and patient safety (Francis, 2013; West et al., 2020).

Aligning leadership, policy and workforce strategies also has implications for *equity and inclusivity*. Research shows that marginalised groups in healthcare – such as women, ethnic minorities and internationally trained staff – experience higher rates of stress, discrimination and career barriers (Begeny et al., 2020; Hall et al., 2016). Leadership, policy and workforce strategies that are aligned around principles of diversity, equity and inclusion (see Buonocore, Scarozza et al., 2025) not only reduce stress among underrepresented groups but also contribute to a more just and resilient healthcare system. For instance, policies that address gender equity in pay and promotion (e.g., Briganti et al., 2023), leadership training that incorporates inclusive practices and workforce strategies that support flexible career paths collectively create environments where all staff can thrive (de Gennaro & Marino, 2024; de Gennaro & Piscopo, 2023).

Finally, alignment must be understood as a *dynamic process* rather than a static achievement. Healthcare environments are constantly evolving due to demographic changes, technological innovations and global crises such as pandemics. Alignment therefore requires ongoing dialogue between leaders, policymakers and frontline professionals, supported by continuous measurement of well-being, patient outcomes and organisational performance. Tools such as staff surveys, patient safety metrics and quality dashboards can provide the data needed to sustain alignment, while participatory governance structures ensure that policies and strategies remain responsive to the realities of clinical practice (West et al., 2018a).

In conclusion, aligning leadership, policy and workforce strategies is both a conceptual necessity and a practical imperative for sustainable healthcare. Fragmentation across these domains perpetuates stress and undermines care, while alignment creates synergy that enhances both staff well-being and patient outcomes. Evidence shows that when leaders are visibly committed, policies are supportive and workforce strategies are robust, healthcare organisations are better equipped to withstand pressures, reduce burnout and deliver high-quality care (Riemma et al., 2025). Ultimately, the path to sustainability lies not in isolated interventions but in the *integration of leadership vision, policy frameworks and workforce strategies* into a coherent system that places well-being and patient care at its core.

7.3 BUILDING SUSTAINABLE AND RESILIENT HEALTHCARE SYSTEMS

The quest for sustainability in healthcare is inseparable from the challenge of building resilience. While sustainability emphasises the long-term capacity of healthcare systems to deliver safe, effective and equitable care without depleting financial, human or environmental resources (World Health Organization, 2016), resilience focuses on the ability of systems to adapt, recover and thrive in the face of shocks, uncertainty and chronic stressors (Hollnagel et al., 2015). Together, these concepts define what it means for healthcare systems not merely to survive but to *flourish under pressure* (Riemma et al., 2025). In an era marked by pandemics, demographic shifts and rising expectations of care, sustainability and resilience are no longer aspirational values; they are strategic necessities.

Healthcare systems around the world have been repeatedly tested by crises, most notably the COVID-19 pandemic, which exposed vulnerabilities in workforce planning, supply chains, leadership and governance (e.g., de Gennaro et al., 2022). At the same time, it revealed the extraordinary adaptive capacities of healthcare organisations when properly supported. Hospitals rapidly reorganised workflows, expanded intensive care capacity and adopted digital technologies to maintain continuity of care (Legido-Quigley et al., 2020). These adaptations, however, came at immense cost to staff well-being, demonstrating that *resilience without sustainability is fragile*. Systems can flex under short-term pressure but eventually falter if long-term investments in workforce, culture and infrastructure are neglected (Maunder et al., 2021).

A sustainable and resilient healthcare system must therefore rest on several interrelated pillars. The first is *workforce sustainability*, which ensures that staffing is sufficient, fairly distributed and supported by policies that prevent burnout and attrition. Research consistently shows that safe staffing ratios and supportive work environments are linked not only to staff retention but also to improved patient outcomes (Aiken et al., 2002; West et al., 2020). Workforce sustainability also entails equity and inclusivity: resilient systems are those in which all professionals – regardless of gender, ethnicity or background – experience fairness, belonging and opportunities for growth (Begeny et al., 2020).

The second pillar is *organisational culture*, particularly cultures that foster psychological safety, compassion and continuous learning. Edmondson (2019) emphasises that organisations capable of learning from failure are those that encourage openness and voice, rather than suppressing error reporting. In healthcare, such cultures reduce stress and enhance patient safety simultaneously (Nembhard & Edmondson, 2006). Compassionate and inclusive leadership practices reinforce these cultural foundations, enabling organisations to support staff in times of stress while maintaining focus on quality and innovation (West et al., 2017).

The third pillar is *systems thinking*, which highlights that resilience is not the product of isolated interventions but emerges from the interconnections between policy, leadership, workforce and technology (Blanchet et al., 2017; Senge, 2006). For example, digital tools that monitor workload and flag risks of burnout are effective only if integrated with supportive leadership and adequate staffing policies. Likewise, policy reforms mandating safe staffing ratios succeed only when leaders translate them into equitable workload management and when workforce strategies ensure sufficient recruitment pipelines. Sustainable resilience therefore requires coherence across levels: micro (teams and individuals), meso (organisations) and macro (health systems and policy).

A fourth pillar is *adaptability and innovation*. Resilient healthcare systems are not static but evolve in response to emerging challenges. The rapid adoption of telehealth during the COVID-19 pandemic illustrates how innovation can simultaneously expand access, reduce pressure on physical facilities and offer new modes of care (Keesara et al., 2020). Yet innovation is sustainable only if it is accompanied by adequate training, investment and evaluation to prevent additional burdens on staff (de Gennaro & Marino, 2024). Too often, digitalisation is introduced without consideration of its impact on workload and well-being, leading to increased stress rather than relief (Agrifoglio & de Gennaro, 2022; Shanafelt et al., 2016). Sustainable systems integrate innovation with human-centred design, ensuring that new technologies enhance rather than undermine resilience.

The fifth pillar is *governance and accountability*. Resilient systems require governance structures that balance flexibility with accountability, enabling rapid adaptation while safeguarding ethical standards and equity (Buonocore, de Gennaro et al., 2025). Transparency in decision-making, inclusive stakeholder engagement and accountability for workforce well-being are essential to building trust and legitimacy (Kruk et al., 2015). Evidence shows that when staff feel their voices are heard in organisational decision-making, stress is reduced and commitment increases (Cummings et al., 2018). Governance that excludes frontline perspectives risks policies that are misaligned with reality, perpetuating stress and inefficiency.

Building sustainable and resilient systems also demands attention to the *interdependence of staff well-being and patient outcomes*. As demonstrated earlier, systems that ignore workforce stress cannot deliver safe or compassionate care. Conversely, systems that invest in staff well-being achieve better clinical outcomes, higher patient satisfaction and lower costs associated with turnover and error (Han et al., 2019; Shanafelt & Noseworthy, 2017). This interdependence makes clear that sustainability is not achieved through financial efficiency alone but through the *integration of human, organisational and clinical dimensions*.

Ultimately, resilience and sustainability are not abstract ideals but practical agendas. They require sustained investment in people, culture and systems; leadership that embodies compassion and accountability; policies that prioritise both workforce and patient needs; and infrastructures that adapt to change without sacrificing equity or safety. The lessons of recent crises highlight both the risks of neglect and the possibilities of reform. Sustainable and resilient healthcare systems are those that emerge stronger from challenges because they treat stress not only as a risk to be minimised but also as an opportunity to reimagine care, strengthen community and align human well-being with the enduring mission of healthcare.

REFERENCES

Agrifoglio, R., & de Gennaro, D. (2022). New ways of working through emerging technologies: A meta-synthesis of the adoption of blockchain in the accountancy domain. *Journal of Theoretical and Applied Electronic*

Commerce Research, *17*, 836–850. ISSN: 0718-1876. https://doi.org/10.3390/jtaer17020043

Aiken, L. H., Clarke, S. P., Sloane, D. M., Sochalski, J., & Silber, J. H. (2002). Hospital nurse staffing and patient mortality, nurse burnout, and job dissatisfaction. *JAMA*, *288*(16), 1987–1993.

Aiken, L. H., Sermeus, W., Van den Heede, K., Sloane, D. M., Busse, R., McKee, M., Bruyneel, L., Rafferty, A. M., Griffiths, P., Moreno-Casbas, M. T., Tishelman, C., Scott, A., Brzostek, T., Kinnunen, J., Schwendimann, R., Heinen, M., Zikos, D., Sjetne, I. S., Smith, H. L., & Kutney-Lee, A. (2012). Patient safety, satisfaction, and quality of hospital care: Cross sectional surveys of nurses and patients in 12 countries in Europe and the United States. *BMJ*, *344*, e1717.

Bakker, A. B., & Demerouti, E. (2007). The Job Demands–Resources model: State of the art. *Journal of Managerial Psychology*, *22*(3), 309–328.

Begeny, C. T., Ryan, M. K., Moss-Racusin, C. A., & Ravetz, G. (2020). In some professions, women have become well represented, yet gender bias persists—a mystery. *Frontiers in Psychology*, *11*, 566.

Blanchet, K., Nam, S. L., Ramalingam, B., & Pozo-Martin, F. (2017). Governance and capacity to manage resilience of health systems: Towards a new conceptual framework. *International Journal of Health Policy and Management*, *6*(8), 431–435.

Briganti, P., de Gennaro, D., Buonocore, F., & Varriale, L. (2023). Job (dis-) satisfaction in pay-for-performance health care contexts: A meta-synthesis of qualitative literature. *International Journal of Public Sector Management*, *36*(6/7), 606–631. https://doi.org/10.1108/IJPSM-02-2023-0061

Buchan, J., Duffield, C., & Jordan, A. (2015). Solving' nursing shortages: Do we need a new agenda? *Journal of Nursing Management*, *23*(5), 543–545.

Buonocore, F., de Gennaro, D., & Del Barone, L. (2025). Ethical and organizational dynamics of non-standard work in public administration: Challenges and opportunities in the digital era. *Personnel Review. ahead-of-print.* https://doi.org/10.1108/PR-05-2024-0506

Buonocore, F., Scarozza, D., de Gennaro, D., & Del Barone, L. (2025). Pathways to diversity management in Italian public administration: The INPS case study. In S. Pulcher, S. Basaglia, S. Cuomo, & Z. Simonella (Eds.), *Diversity and inclusion in Italy: Societal and organizational perspectives* (pp. 231–253). Springer. ISBN: 978-3-031-81937-7. https://doi.org/10.1007/978-3-031-81938-4_11

Cummings, G. G., Tate, K., Lee, S., Wong, C. A., Paananen, T., Micaroni, S. P., & Chatterjee, G. E. (2018). Leadership styles and outcome patterns for the nursing workforce and work environment: A systematic review. *International Journal of Nursing Studies*, *85*, 19–60.

Dall'Ora, C., Ball, J., Reinius, M., & Griffiths, P. (2020). Burnout in nursing: A theoretical review. *Human Resources for Health*, *18*(1), 41.

de Gennaro, D. (2019). Transformational leadership for public service motivation. *Journal of Economic and Administrative Sciences*, *35*(1), 5–15. ISSN: 1026-4116. https://doi.org/10.1108/JEAS-06-2018-0075

de Gennaro, D., Loia, F., & Piscopo, G. (2022). Working role of women in a pandemic world: A poetic inquiry. *Management Research Review*, *45*(11), 1373–1392. ISSN: 2040-8269. https://doi.org/10.1108/MRR-06-2021-0430

de Gennaro, D., & Marino, M. (2024). *Global classroom: Multicultural approaches and organizational strategies in teaching and learning business and economics*. Emerald Publishing Limited. ISBN: 978-1-83549-285-7, eISBN: 978-1-83549-284-0. https://doi.org/10.1108/9781835492840

de Gennaro, D., & Piscopo, G. (2023). Pinkwashing and mansplaining: Experiences of gender inequality at work during the pandemic. *Culture and Organization*, *24*(9), 298–314. ISSN: 1477-2760. https://doi.org/10.1080/14759551.2023.2176501

Del Barone, L., de Gennaro, D., & Buonocore, F. (2025). AI-driven HRM and managerial competencies: Strengthening organizational resilience in Public Administration. *Management Decision. ahead-of-print*. https://doi.org/10.1108/MD-06-2024-1252

Dyrbye, L. N., West, C. P., Sinsky, C. A., Goeders, L. E., Satele, D. V., Tutty, M. A., & Shanafelt, T. D. (2020). Medical licensure questions and physician reluctance to seek care for mental health conditions. *Mayo Clinic Proceedings*, *95*(7), 1486–1493.

Edmondson, A. C. (2019). *The fearless organization: Creating psychological safety in the workplace for learning, innovation, and growth*. Wiley.

Epstein, E. G., & Hamric, A. B. (2009). Moral distress, moral residue, and the crescendo effect. *Journal of Clinical Ethics*, *20*(4), 330–342.

Figley, C. R. (2002). *Compassion fatigue: Psychotherapists' chronic lack of self care*. Brunner-Routledge.

Francis, R. (2013). *Report of the mid staffordshire NHS foundation trust public inquiry*. The Stationery Office.

Gagliarducci, F., & de Gennaro, D. (2020). A project for assessing public management competencies. In M. Decastri, S. Battini, F. Buonocore, & F. Gagliarducci (Eds.), *Organizational development in public administration: The Italian way* (pp. 177–212). Palgrave MacMillan. ISBN: 978-30-30437-98-5. https://doi.org/10.1007/978-3-030-43799-2_6

Griffiths, P., Maruotti, A., Recio Saucedo, A., Redfern, O. C., Ball, J. E., Briggs, J., Dall'Ora, C., Schmidt, P. E., & Smith, G. B. (2020). Nurse staffing, nursing assistants and hospital mortality: Retrospective longitudinal cohort study. *BMJ Quality & Safety*, *28*(8), 609–617.

Hall, L. H., Johnson, J., Watt, I., Tsipa, A., & O'Connor, D. B. (2016). Healthcare staff well-being, burnout, and patient safety: A systematic review. *PLoS One*, *11*(7), e0159015.

Han, S., Shanafelt, T. D., Sinsky, C. A., Awad, K. M., Dyrbye, L. N., Fiscus, L. C., Trockel, M., & Goh, J. (2019). Estimating the attributable cost of physician burnout in the United States. *Annals of Internal Medicine*, *170* (11), 784–790.

Hollnagel, E., Braithwaite, J., & Wears, R. L. (2015). *Resilient health care, volume 2: The resilience of everyday clinical work*. Ashgate.

Jameton, A. (1984). *Nursing practice: The ethical issues*. Prentice-Hall.

Keesara, S., Jonas, A., & Schulman, K. (2020). Covid-19 and health care's digital revolution. *New England Journal of Medicine*, *382*(23), e82.

Kinman, G., & Grant, L. (2020). Presenteeism during the COVID-19 pandemic: Risks and solutions. *Occupational Medicine*, *70*(5), 243–244.

Kruk, M. E., Myers, M., Varpilah, S. T., & Dahn, B. T. (2015). What is a resilient health system? Lessons from Ebola. *The Lancet*, *385*(9980), 1910–1912.

Legido-Quigley, H., Asgari, N., Teo, Y. Y., Leung, G. M., Oshitani, H., Fukuda, K., Cook, A. R., Hsu, L. Y., & Shibuya, K. (2020). Are high-performing health systems resilient against the COVID-19 epidemic? *The Lancet*, *395*(10227), 848–850.

Maunder, R. G., Heeney, N. D., Kiss, A., Hunter, J. J., Jeffs, L., Ginty, L., Wiesenfeld, L., Vytelingum, B., Tannenbaum, D. W., & Mazzulli, T. (2021). Psychological impact of the COVID-19 pandemic on hospital workers over time. *General Hospital Psychiatry, 71*, 88–94.

Nembhard, I. M., & Edmondson, A. C. (2006). Making it safe: The effects of leader inclusiveness and professional status on psychological safety and improvement efforts in health care teams. *Journal of Organizational Behavior, 27*(7), 941–966.

NHS England. (2020). *We are the NHS: People plan for 2020/21 – action for us all.* NHS England.

Panagioti, M., Geraghty, K., Johnson, J., Zhou, A., Panagopoulou, E., Chew-Graham, C., Peters, D., Hodkinson, A., Riley, R., & Esmail, A. (2018). Association between physician burnout and patient safety, professionalism, and patient satisfaction: A systematic review and meta-analysis. *JAMA Internal Medicine, 178*(10), 1317–1330.

Peters, E. (2018). Compassion fatigue in nursing: A concept analysis. *Nursing Forum, 53*(4), 466–480.

Riemma, F., Buonocore, F., & de Gennaro, D. (2025). Coping with pressure: Stress management and organizational support in healthcare settings. *Personnel Review. ahead-of-print.* https://doi.org/10.1108/PR-04-2025-0387

Rushton, C. H. (2018). *Moral resilience: Transforming moral suffering in healthcare.* Oxford University Press.

Schaufeli, W. B., & Bakker, A. B. (2004). Job demands, job resources, and their relationship with burnout and engagement: A multi-sample study. *Journal of Organizational Behavior, 25*(3), 293–315.

Senge, P. M. (2006). *The fifth discipline: The art & practice of the learning organization.* Doubleday.

Shanafelt, T. D., Dyrbye, L. N., Sinsky, C., & West, C. P. (2016). Addressing physician burnout: The way forward. *JAMA, 317*(9), 901–902.

Shanafelt, T. D., Goh, J., & Sinsky, C. (2017). The business case for investing in physician well-being. *JAMA Internal Medicine, 177*(12), 1826–1832.

Shanafelt, T. D., & Noseworthy, J. H. (2017). Executive leadership and physician well-being: Nine organizational strategies to promote engagement and reduce burnout. *Mayo Clinic Proceedings*, *92*(1), 129–146.

Swensen, S., Kabcenell, A., & Shanafelt, T. (2016). Physician–organization collaboration reduces physician burnout and promotes engagement: The Mayo Clinic experience. *Journal of Healthcare Management*, *61*(2), 105–127.

Tawfik, D. S., Profit, J., Morgenthaler, T. I., Satele, D. V., Sinsky, C. A., Dyrbye, L. N., Tutty, M. A., West, C. P., & Shanafelt, T. D. (2019). Physician burnout, well-being, and work unit safety grades in relation to reported medical errors. *Mayo Clinic Proceedings*, *94*(11), 2025–2036.

West, M., Bailey, S., & Williams, E. (2020). *The courage of compassion: Supporting nurses and midwives to deliver high-quality care*. The King's Fund.

West, C. P., Dyrbye, L. N., & Shanafelt, T. D. (2018a). Physician burnout: Contributors, consequences and solutions. *Journal of Internal Medicine*, *283*(6), 516–529.

West, C. P., Dyrbye, L. N., & Shanafelt, T. D. (2018b). Interventions to prevent and reduce physician burnout: A systematic review and meta-analysis. *The Lancet*, *388*(10057), 2272–2281.

West, M., Eckert, R., Collins, B., & Chowla, R. (2017). *Caring to change: How compassionate leadership can stimulate innovation in health care*. The King's Fund.

World Health Organization. (2016). *Global strategy on human resources for health: Workforce 2030*. WHO.

8

A CALL TO ACTION

ABSTRACT

This concluding chapter issues a call to action by translating the book's theoretical and empirical insights into concrete guidance for managers, policymakers and healthcare professionals. It argues that stress in healthcare is an immediate and systemic challenge that demands action at multiple levels, rather than a problem to be deferred to long-term reform alone. This chapter emphasises that meaningful improvements in well-being and patient care can begin today through leadership behaviours, policy choices and professional practices that acknowledge stress as a collective and organisational responsibility.

This chapter outlines actionable steps for organisational leaders, including recognising well-being as a strategic priority, ensuring fair workload distribution, strengthening peer support and creating visible forums for listening and reflection. For policymakers, it highlights the importance of safe staffing standards, reduced bureaucratic burden, ethical clarity and the integration of workforce well-being into quality and safety frameworks. For healthcare professionals, it acknowledges the value of individual and collective coping practices while emphasising the importance of collective voice and advocacy to drive systemic change.

Looking beyond immediate actions, this chapter examines three long-term challenges shaping healthcare work, demographic change, digital transformation and recurring global health crises and shows how their interaction intensifies stress if not proactively addressed through human-centred and system-based strategies. It concludes by arguing that sustainable and resilient healthcare requires a renewed social and organisational compact, aligning leadership, policy, workforce strategies and professional values to transform stress from a corrosive force into a driver of renewal, innovation and humane care.

Keywords: Call to action; healthcare workforce well-being; policy and leadership alignment; healthcare sustainability; future of healthcare work

8.1 WHAT MANAGERS, POLICYMAKERS AND PROFESSIONALS CAN DO TODAY

The evidence presented throughout this book makes clear that stress in healthcare is not an abstract phenomenon or a distant threat: it is a present and pressing reality. The weight of empirical research and practical experience shows that unmanaged stress erodes the well-being of healthcare professionals, undermines patient safety and compromises organisational sustainability. While long-term reforms are necessary to build sustainable and resilient healthcare systems, there is also an urgent need for *immediate action*. Managers, policymakers and professionals at all levels can take meaningful steps today to reduce stress, foster resilience and align the dual goals of staff well-being and patient care. These actions may not solve every systemic problem, but they represent concrete interventions that can create momentum for wider change.

For *managers and organisational leaders*, the most immediate task is to recognise staff well-being as a strategic priority, not a peripheral concern. Evidence shows that when leaders visibly endorse and act on well-being initiatives, staff are more likely to engage with them and less likely to perceive them as tokenistic (Shanafelt & Noseworthy, 2017). Leaders can begin by ensuring equitable workload distribution, supporting flexible scheduling and actively soliciting feedback from staff about stressors in their daily work. Practices such as 'leader rounding,' where managers spend time in clinical areas listening to staff concerns, have been shown to reduce stress and increase trust (Studer, 2003). Small but symbolic actions – such as publicly recognising staff contributions or ensuring rest areas are respected – signal that leadership values the humanity of its workforce.

Managers can also immediately strengthen *peer support and reflective practice*. Programmes like Schwartz Rounds, which provide safe spaces for staff to share the emotional challenges of care, have been shown to reduce isolation and increase empathy across teams (Maben et al., 2018). Similarly, developing or expanding peer support networks ensures that clinicians experiencing distress – especially after adverse events – have immediate access to colleagues who understand their challenges (Hu et al., 2012; Shapiro & Galowitz, 2016). These interventions require minimal infrastructure and can be implemented quickly, yet they have profound effects on reducing stress and fostering collective resilience.

For *policymakers*, immediate steps can be taken to reduce systemic stressors by providing clear mandates and supportive frameworks. Research shows that safe staffing legislation, such as the nurse-to-patient ratio laws in California, directly reduces stress among staff while improving patient outcomes (Aiken et al., 2010). While systemic workforce reforms take time, policymakers can act today by committing to minimum staffing standards, providing emergency funding to alleviate critical shortages and protecting time for professional development. Moreover, policies that explicitly address staff well-being – such as including well-being metrics in quality and safety frameworks – send a powerful signal that workforce sustainability is a core element of healthcare quality (NHS England, 2020). Even incremental policy adjustments, such as reducing bureaucratic reporting requirements or streamlining electronic documentation systems, can immediately reduce administrative burden and give professionals more time for patient care (Shanafelt et al., 2016).

Policymakers can also enhance well-being by embedding *ethical clarity and moral support* into regulations. Moral distress is one of the most pervasive stressors in healthcare, arising when professionals are constrained from providing the care they believe is right (Epstein & Hamric, 2009). By issuing clear guidelines, ensuring transparency in rationing decisions and supporting ethics consultation services, policymakers can help reduce the burden of moral conflict. These measures can be introduced relatively quickly and provide immediate relief for professionals navigating ethically challenging environments.

For *healthcare professionals themselves*, immediate steps are also possible, though the burden of systemic reform should not rest solely on their shoulders. Evidence suggests that individual practices such as mindfulness, reflective writing and structured recovery periods can help mitigate stress in the short term (Spinelli et al., 2019; West et al., 2016). Participation in peer support programmes, mentorship relationships or team debriefings can also enhance resilience and reduce feelings of isolation. Importantly, professionals can advocate collectively – through professional associations, unions and quality improvement initiatives – for organisational and policy changes that align with their lived experiences. Research shows that when staff voices are included in decision-making, organisational strategies are more effective and sustainable (Nembhard & Edmondson, 2006).

A central theme across all levels of action is the need to *move beyond rhetoric to accountability*. Managers can measure staff well-being as routinely as they measure patient outcomes; policymakers can include workforce sustainability indicators in national quality frameworks; and professionals can hold leadership accountable through active participation in governance. Immediate actions such as administering well-being surveys, creating feedback loops and publishing workforce indicators send a strong signal that well-being is not optional but integral to healthcare quality (West et al., 2020).

What can be done today, therefore, is not trivial. Leaders can listen and respond, policymakers can legislate and support and professionals can engage and advocate. These steps do not require waiting for long-term structural reform – they can be enacted immediately, creating the conditions for broader change to follow. Moreover, early interventions create visible improvements in morale, trust and engagement, which in turn strengthen the credibility of larger reform agendas. By acting now, managers, policymakers and professionals can begin to shift healthcare systems from a state of crisis management towards a trajectory of sustainability and resilience.

8.2 LONG-TERM CHALLENGES: DEMOGRAPHICS, DIGITALISATION, GLOBAL HEALTH CRISES

While managers, policymakers and professionals can act today to reduce stress and enhance resilience, the sustainability of healthcare systems ultimately depends on how they prepare for and respond to long-term challenges. Three dynamics in particular – demographic change, digital transformation and recurring global health crises – are poised to shape the landscape of healthcare work for decades to come. These forces are not distant possibilities but unfolding realities that intersect with each other in complex ways. Understanding and addressing them is essential for building resilient and sustainable healthcare systems that protect both staff well-being and patient care.

8.2.1 Demographic Change

Demographic pressures affect both the supply and demand sides of healthcare. On the demand side, ageing populations across much of the world are driving unprecedented increases in chronic disease, multi-morbidity and long-term care needs (World Health Organization, 2015). The Organisation for Economic Co-operation and Development (OECD) has increasingly emphasised the importance of strengthening health systems and supporting the well-being of healthcare professionals (OECD, 2019). These pressures translate into heavier workloads, more complex clinical cases and heightened emotional demands for healthcare professionals, who must manage the challenges of prolonged patient trajectories and end-of-life care (Riemma et al., 2025). On the supply side, healthcare workforces themselves are ageing. The World Health Organization (2020) estimates that one in six nurses worldwide will retire within the next decade, intensifying shortages that are already acute. Without proactive workforce planning – through investment in training, international mobility frameworks and retention strategies – healthcare systems risk entering a vicious cycle of escalating demand and shrinking supply (Buchan et al., 2015).

8.2.2 Digitalisation

Digital transformation is often presented as the solution to healthcare's structural challenges, but its implications for staff well-being and patient care are deeply ambivalent. On one hand, digital tools promise greater efficiency, enhanced data analytics and new modalities of care. Telemedicine, for example, expanded dramatically during the COVID-19 pandemic, improving access for patients and reducing exposure risks for staff (Keesara et al., 2020). Artificial intelligence and predictive analytics are increasingly used to support diagnostics, workflow optimisation and population health management (Topol, 2019). Electronic health records (EHRs) have the potential to improve coordination and continuity of care.

On the other hand, digitalisation can exacerbate stress if poorly implemented (Agrifoglio & de Gennaro, 2022). Research shows that EHR systems often increase clerical burden, reduce time available for direct patient care and contribute to physician burnout (Shanafelt et al., 2016). Algorithmic decision-making may undermine professional autonomy if not transparently integrated into clinical judgement (Greenhalgh et al., 2019). Moreover, digital inequities risk reinforcing disparities in both patient access and workforce capacity, as under-resourced organisations may lack the infrastructure or training to benefit fully from new technologies (van Dijk, 2020). For digitalisation to contribute to sustainability rather than stress, it must be human-centred, co-designed with professionals and implemented alongside organisational changes that preserve autonomy and reduce administrative burden (Buonocore et al., 2024).

8.2.3 Global Health Crises

The COVID-19 pandemic highlighted with devastating clarity that healthcare systems are only as strong as their weakest links. The pandemic produced unprecedented levels of stress among healthcare professionals, with global surveys reporting burnout rates exceeding 50% in many contexts (Kisely et al., 2020; Maunder et al., 2021). While the pandemic was extraordinary in scale, global health crises are likely to recur, whether in the form of infectious disease outbreaks, climate-related disasters or geopolitical instability (Patel et al., 2020). Each crisis exacerbates existing vulnerabilities – workforce shortages, supply chain fragility, inequities in access – and places extraordinary demands on healthcare staff (de Gennaro et al., 2022).

The lessons of COVID-19 are clear: reactive crisis management is insufficient. Building resilience requires sustained investment in surge capacity, protective infrastructure and psychosocial support for staff (Legido-Quigley et al., 2020). Importantly, crisis preparedness must explicitly include workforce well-being as a strategic priority. Evidence from the pandemic shows that organisations that provided transparent communication, psychological support and flexible redeployment strategies fared better in protecting staff from extreme distress (Greenberg et al., 2020). Policymakers must therefore institutionalise support mechanisms – such as rapid-response mental health teams and protected rest periods – so that they are not improvised in the midst of crisis but embedded into standard preparedness frameworks.

These long-term challenges – demographic pressures, digital transformation and global crises – are deeply interconnected. An ageing population increases demand for care just as workforce retirements reduce supply. Digitalisation may mitigate these pressures by enabling new models of care, but it also risks adding to stress if poorly integrated. Global crises then stress-test these fragile dynamics, amplifying vulnerabilities and exposing systemic weaknesses. The implication is clear: sustainability and resilience require not only addressing each challenge in isolation but also recognising and managing their intersections. For example, investment in digital technologies must be accompanied by workforce training and ethical safeguards (D'Avino et al., 2024); demographic shifts must be addressed through both workforce expansion and new care models; and crisis preparedness must link supply chain management with staff support systems.

In short, healthcare systems must adopt a *foresight-oriented, systems-based approach* that anticipates these long-term challenges and integrates responses across leadership, policy and workforce domains. Demographics, digitalisation and global crises are not temporary stressors to be endured but structural features of the healthcare landscape. By embedding these realities into strategic planning today, managers, policymakers and professionals can move from reactive coping to proactive transformation, ensuring that healthcare systems remain not only sustainable but also humane in the decades to come.

8.3 THE FUTURE OF WORK AND CARE IN HEALTHCARE

Looking to the future, it is evident that healthcare work will not return to a mythical equilibrium in which stress is a marginal or temporary concern. Instead, stress will remain a central feature of the profession, shaped by technological innovation, demographic change and global crises. The challenge is therefore not to eliminate stress – an impossible goal – but to redesign healthcare systems so that stress does not erode well-being, professional integrity or patient safety. The future of work and care in healthcare must be understood as a dynamic interplay between evolving workforce expectations, new models of care and emerging societal demands.

The evolving workforce. One of the most striking trends is the transformation of workforce expectations. New generations of healthcare professionals are less willing to accept chronic overwork, hierarchical cultures and poor work–life balance as inevitable conditions of the job (see de Gennaro et al., 2023 for a focus on Generation Z workforce). Surveys consistently show that younger clinicians prioritise flexibility, autonomy and meaningful work, even more than financial reward (Twenge et al., 2010). This generational shift has the potential to reshape organisational cultures (see Annosi et al., 2025): employers that fail to adapt may struggle with recruitment and retention, while those that embrace flexible scheduling, participatory governance and inclusive leadership will be better positioned to attract and retain talent. The future of healthcare work will therefore be influenced not only by demographic shortages but also by changing social norms around what constitutes acceptable and sustainable employment.

New models of care. The organisation of healthcare delivery is also shifting towards models that are more integrated, team-based and community-oriented. The rise of multidisciplinary teams, community health workers and integrated care pathways reflects recognition that fragmented care is inefficient, stressful and unsafe (Valentijn et al., 2013). Interprofessional collaboration reduces duplication, enhances continuity and distributes stress across teams rather than concentrating it on individual clinicians. Research suggests that integrated care models are associated with better patient outcomes and higher job satisfaction for staff, as they align professional practice with holistic visions of care (Reeves et al., 2017). In the future, healthcare will likely move further in this direction, with teams that include not only physicians and nurses but also digital health specialists, social workers and patient advocates. This expansion of roles offers opportunities to distribute workload and reduce stress but also requires strong leadership, clear role definitions and shared values to prevent conflict and role ambiguity.

Digital transformation and the hybridisation of work. Digitalisation will profoundly shape the future of healthcare work. Telemedicine, remote monitoring and artificial intelligence will increasingly redefine the boundaries of care, enabling professionals to deliver services across space and time (Topol, 2019). For staff, this shift presents both opportunities and risks. On one hand, digital tools can reduce physical workload, expand access to expertise and allow more flexible work arrangements (Keesara et al., 2020). On the other hand, poorly designed digital systems risk intensifying administrative burden, eroding professional autonomy and blurring the boundaries between work and personal life (Agrifoglio & de Gennaro, 2022; Shanafelt et al., 2016). The challenge for the future is to ensure that digital transformation is guided by human-centred design principles, co-created with professionals and evaluated not only for efficiency but also for its impact on staff well-being and patient relationships (Greenhalgh et al., 2017).

Globalisation and interconnected vulnerability. The future of healthcare is also global. Pandemics, climate change, migration and geopolitical instability will increasingly shape local healthcare realities. The COVID-19 pandemic demonstrated how quickly global crises cascade into local stress for frontline staff (Legido-Quigley et al., 2020). Climate-related health impacts – heatwaves, vector-borne diseases, air pollution – will further strain systems already under pressure (Watts et al., 2019). These challenges highlight the need for transnational collaboration in workforce planning, data sharing and crisis preparedness. Healthcare professionals will need to develop not only clinical skills but also competencies in adaptability, cross-cultural communication and ethical decision-making under uncertainty (Kickbusch et al., 2016).

Professional identity and meaning. Perhaps the most profound question for the future of healthcare work is how professionals will sustain meaning and identity in environments of constant pressure (Riemma et al., 2025). Research shows that meaningful work is a key determinant of resilience, engagement and patient-centred care (Rosso et al., 2010). Yet when organisational conditions undermine values – through bureaucratic overload, inadequate recognition or moral compromise – meaning is eroded, leading to burnout and attrition (Grace & VanHeuvelen, 2019). The future of care will therefore depend on organisations' ability to nurture moral and vocational dimensions of work, ensuring that professionals can connect their daily labour with broader purposes of healing, compassion and justice. Initiatives that support reflective practice, professional development and recognition of moral complexity will be central to sustaining professional integrity in the decades to come.

Towards resilient, humane healthcare. Bringing these strands together, the future of healthcare work requires a new compact between organisations, policymakers and professionals. This compact must acknowledge that staff well-being and patient care are inseparable, that sustainability demands both workforce planning and cultural change and that resilience is collective rather than individual. Healthcare systems must move away from models that valorise sacrifice and stoicism and towards models that institutionalise support, recognition and shared responsibility. The healthcare systems that thrive in the future will be those that integrate technological innovation with human-centred design, global preparedness with local compassion and professional identity with organisational sustainability.

In conclusion, the future of work and care in healthcare will be defined by its ability to reconcile enduring pressures with emerging possibilities. Stress will remain, but it need not be destructive. With thoughtful leadership, supportive policies, robust workforce strategies and an unwavering commitment to the moral and human dimensions of care, healthcare systems can transform stress from a corrosive force into a catalyst for innovation, solidarity and renewal. The ultimate challenge is not merely to adapt to the future but to shape it – creating healthcare systems that are not only resilient and sustainable but also humane, just and worthy of the professionals and patients who depend on them.

REFERENCES

Agrifoglio, R., & de Gennaro, D. (2022). New ways of working through emerging technologies: A meta-synthesis of the adoption of blockchain in the accountancy domain. *Journal of Theoretical and Applied Electronic Commerce Research*, *17*, 836–850. ISSN: 0718-1876. https://doi.org/10.3390/jtaer17020043

Aiken, L. H., Sloane, D. M., Cimiotti, J. P., Clarke, S. P., Flynn, L., Seago, J. A., Spetz, J., & Smith, H. L. (2010). Implications of the California nurse staffing mandate for other states. *Health Services Research*, *45*(4), 904–921.

Annosi, M. C., Hughes, M., de Gennaro, D., Oppedisano, R., & Buonocore, F. (2025). Bridging generations: Managing cognitive conflicts during technology adoption in multigenerational family firms. *Journal of Family Business Strategy*. ahead-of-print.

Buchan, J., Duffield, C., & Jordan, A. (2015). Solving' nursing shortages: Do we need a new agenda? *Journal of Nursing Management*, *23*(5), 543–545.

Buonocore, F., Annosi, M. C., de Gennaro, D., & Riemma, F. (2024). Digital transformation and social change: Leadership strategies for responsible innovation. *Journal of Engineering and Technology Management*, *74*, 1–14. https://doi.org/10.1016/j.jengtecman.2024.101843

D'Avino, E., de Gennaro, D., Inno, L., & Vicentini, G. (2024). Promoting equality through ethical AI and DEI principles: A case study of the LSST. In D. de Gennaro & M. Marino (Eds.), *Global classroom: Multicultural approaches and organizational strategies in teaching and learning business and economics* (pp. 161–166). Emerald Publishing Limited. ISBN: 978-1-83549-285-7. https://doi.org/10.1108/978-1-83549-284-020241020

de Gennaro, D., Loia, F., & Piscopo, G. (2022). Working role of women in a pandemic world: A poetic inquiry. *Management Research Review*, *45*(11), 1373–1392. ISSN: 2040-8269. https://doi.org/10.1108/MRR-06-2021-0430

de Gennaro, D., Mormile, S., Piscopo, G., & Adinolfi, P. (2023). In the jungle, the mighty jungle, the zebras are teal tonight: Investigating the organizational forms of generation Z-driven Italian start-ups. *Journal of Small Business and Enterprise Development*, *30*(6), 1129–1155. ISSN: 1462-6004. https://doi.org/10.1108/JSBED-02-2023-0063

Epstein, E. G., & Hamric, A. B. (2009). Moral distress, moral residue, and the crescendo effect. *Journal of Clinical Ethics*, *20*(4), 330–342.

Grace, P. J., & VanHeuvelen, J. S. (2019). Occupational identity and moral distress in critical care nurses. *Nursing Ethics*, *26*(4), 1191–1205.

Greenberg, N., Docherty, M., Gnanapragasam, S., & Wessely, S. (2020). Managing mental health challenges faced by healthcare workers during COVID-19. *BMJ*, *368*, m1211.

Greenhalgh, T., Wherton, J., Papoutsi, C., Lynch, J., & Hughes, G. (2017). Beyond adoption: A new framework for theorizing and evaluating nonadoption, abandonment, and challenges to the scale-up, spread, and sustainability of health and care technologies. *Journal of Medical Internet Research*, *19*(11), e367.

Greenhalgh, T., Wherton, J., Papoutsi, C., Lynch, J., & Hughes, G. (2019). Infrastructure revisited: An ethnographic case study of how health information infrastructure shapes and constrains technological innovation. *Journal of Medical Internet Research*, *21*(12), e16093.

Hu, Y. Y., Fix, M. L., Hevelone, N. D., Lipsitz, S. R., Greenberg, C. C., & Shapiro, J. (2012). Physicians' needs in coping with emotional stressors: The case for peer support. *Archives of Surgery*, *147*(3), 212–217.

Keesara, S., Jonas, A., & Schulman, K. (2020). Covid-19 and health care's digital revolution. *New England Journal of Medicine*, *382*(23), e82.

Kickbusch, I., Franz, C., & Medcalf, L. (2016). Global health diplomacy: Training across disciplines. *Bulletin of the World Health Organization*, *94* (5), 356–356A.

Kisely, S., Warren, N., McMahon, L., Dalais, C., Henry, I., & Siskind, D. (2020). Occurrence, prevention, and management of the psychological effects of emerging virus outbreaks on healthcare workers: Rapid review and meta-analysis. *BMJ*, *369*, m1642.

Legido-Quigley, H., Asgari, N., Teo, Y. Y., Leung, G. M., Oshitani, H., Fukuda, K., Cook, A. R., Hsu, L. Y., & Shibuya, K. (2020). Are high-performing health systems resilient against the COVID-19 epidemic? *The Lancet*, *395*(10227), 848–850.

Maben, J., Bridges, J., Adams, M., Peccei, R., Murrells, T., & Robert, G. (2018). Recognising and rewarding compassionate care: Exploring the implications of the Francis report for nurse education and practice. *Journal of Nursing Management*, *26*(4).

Maunder, R. G., Heeney, N. D., Kiss, A., Hunter, J. J., Jeffs, L., Ginty, L., Wiesenfeld, L., Vytelingum, B., Tannenbaum, D. W., & Mazzulli, T. (2021). Psychological impact of the COVID-19 pandemic on hospital workers over time. *General Hospital Psychiatry*, *71*, 88–94.

Nembhard, I. M., & Edmondson, A. C. (2006). Making it safe: The effects of leader inclusiveness and professional status on psychological safety and improvement efforts in health care teams. *Journal of Organizational Behavior*, *27*(7), 941–966.

NHS England. (2020). *We are the NHS: People plan for 2020/21 – action for us all.* NHS England.

OECD. (2019). *Health at a Glance 2019: OECD indicators*. OECD Publishing.

Patel, S. S., Rogers, M. B., Amlôt, R., & Rubin, G. J. (2020). What do we mean by "community resilience"? A systematic literature review of how it is defined in the literature. *PLoS Currents*, *9*.

Reeves, S., Pelone, F., Harrison, R., Goldman, J., & Zwarenstein, M. (2017). Interprofessional collaboration to improve professional practice and healthcare outcomes. *Cochrane Database of Systematic Reviews*, *6*, CD000072.

Riemma, F., Buonocore, F., & de Gennaro, D. (2025). Coping with pressure: Stress management and organizational support in healthcare settings. *Personnel Review. ahead-of-print.* https://doi.org/10.1108/PR-04-2025-0387

Rosso, B. D., Dekas, K. H., & Wrzesniewski, A. (2010). On the meaning of work: A theoretical integration and review. *Research in Organizational Behavior*, *30*, 91–127.

Shanafelt, T. D., Dyrbye, L. N., & West, C. P., (2016). Addressing physician burnout: The way forward. *JAMA*, *317*(9), 901–902.

Shanafelt, T. D., & Noseworthy, J. H. (2017). Executive leadership and physician well-being: Nine organizational strategies to promote engagement and reduce burnout. *Mayo Clinic Proceedings*, *92*(1), 129–146.

Shapiro, J., & Galowitz, P. (2016). Peer support for clinicians: A programmatic approach. *Academic Medicine*, *91*(9), 1200–1204.

Spinelli, C., Wisener, M., & Khoury, B. (2019). Mindfulness training for healthcare professionals and trainees: A meta-analysis of randomized controlled trials. *Journal of Psychosomatic Research*, *120*, 29–38.

Studer, Q. (2003). *Hardwiring excellence: Purpose, worthwhile work, making a difference*. Fire Starter Publishing.

Topol, E. (2019). *Deep medicine: How artificial intelligence can make healthcare human again*. Basic Books.

Twenge, J. M., Campbell, S. M., Hoffman, B. J., & Lance, C. E. (2010). Generational differences in work values: Leisure and extrinsic values increasing, social and intrinsic values decreasing. *Journal of Management*, *36*(5), 1117–1142.

Valentijn, P. P., Schepman, S. M., Opheij, W., & Bruijnzeels, M. A. (2013). Understanding integrated care: A comprehensive conceptual framework based on the integrative functions of primary care. *International Journal of Integrated Care*, *13*, e010.

van Dijk, J. A. G. M. (2020). *The digital divide*. Polity Press.

Watts, R., Bowles, D., Fisher, C., & Li, I. (2019). Meaningful recognition programmes and the impact on healthcare staff well-being. *Journal of Nursing Management*, *27*(6), 1172–1180.

West, M., Bailey, S., & Williams, E. (2020). *The courage of compassion: Supporting nurses and midwives to deliver high-quality care*. The King's Fund.

West, C. P., Dyrbye, L. N., Erwin, P. J., & Shanafelt, T. D. (2016). Interventions to prevent and reduce physician burnout: A systematic review and meta-analysis. *The Lancet*, *388*(10057), 2272–2281.

World Health Organization. (2015). *World report on ageing and health*. WHO.

World Health Organization. (2020). *State of the World's nursing 2020: Investing in education, jobs and leadership*. WHO.

CONCLUSION

This book set out to explore one of the most pressing challenges of contemporary healthcare: the pervasive and enduring stress experienced by professionals and the organisational conditions that either mitigate or exacerbate its effects. What began as a recognition of stress as a critical occupational hazard has developed into a more comprehensive understanding of stress as a *systemic feature of healthcare work* – not simply an individual problem to be solved, but a complex, multi-level phenomenon that affects professionals, patients and organisations alike.

In *Part I*, we examined the growing pressure on healthcare professionals, situating stress within the broader dynamics of healthcare as a uniquely high-pressure environment. We traced how global crises, most notably COVID-19, intensified existing vulnerabilities and revealed that stress is not an episodic disruption but a chronic reality. The analysis highlighted the *consequences of stress across three domains*: for professionals, leading to burnout, attrition and moral distress; for patients, manifesting in reduced safety, lower satisfaction and compromised outcomes; and for organisations, resulting in diminished resilience, higher turnover costs and threats to sustainability. Stress, we concluded, is both a human and systemic concern – eroding not only the well-being of those who provide care but also the very quality of the care delivered.

Part II turned to the theoretical frameworks that help us understand and interpret stress. Classic models – the Transactional Model of Stress and Coping, the Demand–Control Model and the Effort–Reward Imbalance Model – were shown to provide important insights into the dynamics of appraisal, control and recognition. Yet healthcare also pushes these models to evolve. The discussion of resilience and the Job Demands–Resources (JD-R) framework underscored the need to integrate resources – social, structural and cultural – into stress theories. Healthcare demonstrates with particular clarity that stress cannot be understood solely as an individual appraisal of demands but must be analysed within the *collective, organisational and systemic contexts* where it occurs.

In *Part III*, we expanded these models by integrating findings from healthcare research into broader theories of stress. The central insight was that resilience must be understood not as an individual trait but as a *collective capacity* sustained by teams, cultures and organisations. Healthcare adds unique dimensions to general stress theories – emotional labour, moral distress, interprofessional dynamics and systemic constraints – that enrich our conceptual frameworks. These sector-specific insights challenge the individualising rhetoric that too often dominates stress discourse and instead emphasise the *responsibility of organisations* to create environments that enable adaptive responses, protect moral integrity and sustain meaningful work.

Part IV asked what it means to move from crisis to sustainability. We argued that staff well-being and patient care are not competing priorities but two sides of the same coin. Sustainable healthcare systems recognise their interdependence and design policies, leadership strategies and workforce planning accordingly. Alignment across these domains – leadership vision, supportive policy and robust workforce strategies – was shown to be a key determinant of resilience. Without such alignment, interventions remain fragmented and ineffective; with alignment, they create virtuous cycles that reinforce both staff engagement and patient outcomes.

Looking to the future, we examined three long-term challenges that will shape healthcare work: demographics, digitalisation and global health crises. Each presents profound risks but also opportunities for innovation and renewal. An ageing population demands new care models and workforce strategies; digitalisation offers potential for efficiency and access but must be human-centred to avoid adding stress; global crises will recur, making preparedness, adaptability and psychosocial support essential. The future of healthcare work, we concluded, will depend on systems' ability to integrate these dynamics while sustaining the moral and vocational dimensions of professional practice.

Several core messages emerge across the book:

- *Stress is systemic.* It is generated not only by individual demands but also by organisational structures, cultural norms and policy environments. Treating stress as an individual failing or weakness obscures the systemic drivers that must be addressed.

- *Well-being and patient care are inseparable.* Evidence consistently shows that the conditions under which staff work shape the quality of care patients receive. Investing in staff well-being is therefore not optional but integral to patient safety and organisational performance.

- *Resilience is collective.* The capacity to adapt to stress emerges from teams, cultures and systems – not only from individual coping strategies. Organisational support, leadership and alignment are critical to sustaining resilience.
- *Leadership matters.* Leadership styles and practices directly influence stress, burnout and engagement. Compassionate, authentic and inclusive leadership reduces stress and fosters environments where professionals can thrive.
- *Alignment is essential.* Policies, leadership practices and workforce strategies must be integrated. Fragmentation across these domains perpetuates stress, while alignment creates the conditions for sustainable resilience.
- *The future demands foresight.* Demographics, digitalisation and global crises will define the healthcare landscape. Addressing these challenges requires proactive, systems-based strategies that embed staff well-being into the core of healthcare design.

For *research*, the insights from healthcare suggest the need to move beyond individual-level models of stress to frameworks that incorporate organisational, systemic and ethical dimensions. Future research should integrate patient outcomes into stress theories, explore collective resilience processes and evaluate interventions at multiple levels of the system.

For *policy*, the message is clear: workforce sustainability must be treated as a cornerstone of healthcare quality. Policymakers should mandate safe staffing levels, fund professional development and include well-being indicators in national quality frameworks. Policies must also address equity, ensuring that marginalised groups in healthcare experience fairness, inclusion and recognition.

For *practice*, managers and leaders must act today to create supportive environments: listening to staff, redistributing workload, implementing peer support and recognising contributions. These practical interventions, though often small, are powerful signals that well-being is valued. More broadly, leaders must embed well-being into organisational strategy, measure it regularly and hold themselves accountable for outcomes.

The conclusions of this book point not to despair but to possibility. Stress in healthcare is real, persistent and damaging, but it is also *malleable*. The evidence shows that when organisations invest in people, when policies prioritise sustainability, and when leaders embody compassion and accountability, stress can be transformed from a corrosive force into a catalyst for learning, solidarity and innovation.

The future of healthcare depends on recognising that the well-being of professionals and the care of patients are intertwined. To ignore this reality is to risk systems that are efficient on paper but unsustainable in practice. To embrace it is to create healthcare systems that are resilient, humane and just – worthy of both those who provide care and those who receive it.

The task ahead is not easy. It demands courage from policymakers, vision from leaders, commitment from organisations and resilience from professionals. But it also offers an opportunity: to reshape healthcare in ways that honour the dignity of work, protect the humanity of professionals and safeguard the health of patients. In this sense, the story of stress in healthcare is not only a story of pressure and burden – it is also a story of resilience, renewal and hope.

INDEX

Printed and bound by CPI Group (UK) Ltd, Croydon, CR0 4YY
14/09/2026
14961562-0007